INTERMITTENT F̶ WOMEN OV̶

Accelerate Weight Loss and Boost Your Energy with this Step-by-Step Guide that Will Turn Back the Clock | 60 Tasty Recipes and a 21-Day Meal Plan Included

Chloe Cooper

Table of Contents

Introduction

Before we officially begin, I would like to thank you for purchasing this book, Intermittent Fasting for Women Over 50.

Feeling a little sluggish lately? Dropping those dress sizes just isn't as easy as it used to be? Have you considered a new way of eating called intermittent fasting? Intermittent fasting, or IF, is one of the most effective ways to lose weight quickly and improve your overall health.

What Is Intermittent Fasting and How Does It Work?

Intermittent fasting is an umbrella term that includes several different diet protocols. Most common intermittent fasts involve including periods of prolonged caloric restriction on an infrequent schedule (e.g., alternate day, every other day). This could be achieved by eating only 500 calories two days per week, for example. Another common variation involves restricting calories all seven days of the week with the exception of one "cheat day" or meal every week. The idea is to alternate periods of fasting and feeding, which can have a number of health benefits.

Intermittent fasting can improve health and longevity by mimicking the effects of calorie restriction, allowing your body to shift from burning sugar to burning stored fat for energy, as occurs during starvation. In other words, intermittent fasting causes your body to burn fat in between meals instead of burning only sugar from eating food. You may already do this naturally by skipping breakfast or snacking only here and there throughout the day. This type of routine is known as "Intermittent Energy Restriction" (IER). Many athletes and health professionals are incorporating this type of eating schedule as a way to shed pounds and improve overall health.

What Is the Variance Between Intermittent Fasting and Calorie Restriction?

Calorie restriction has been shown to reduce the risk of many diseases, including heart disease, stroke, Type II diabetes, cancer, and Alzheimer's disease. Calorie restriction involves reducing daily calorie intake by 20-40% while making sure to consume all essential nutrients. Intermittent fasting incorporates prolonged caloric restriction on an infrequent schedule (e.g., alternate day, every other day). This can be attained by consumption of only 500 calories two days per week, for example. Remember that your body receives less than 20% of its total calories from food; the remaining 80% comes from stored energy reserves (e.g., fat). So, when you fast, your body is forced to burn the fat in your reserves for energy.

Calorie restriction has been shown to have life-extending properties. One study at the University of Wisconsin found that restricting calories by 30% led to a nearly 50% increase in life span in worms! Other studies suggest that calorie restriction may decrease rates of cancer and reduce symptoms such as arthritis and dementia.

While calorie restriction is not necessarily easier than intermittent fasting, it has been around longer and is considered the gold standard when it comes to dieting protocols. For many people, it may be easier to stick with a simple calorie restriction diet, since all you have to do is cut back on your food intake. Intermittent fasting may take a bit more effort and will most likely require an adjustment period.

Some research suggests that intermittent fasting could be as effective as calorie restriction at promoting weight loss while improving overall health and longevity. Research in mice with liver cancer demonstrates that IF could be used to control the progression of the disease. IF has also been shown to decrease body weight and insulin levels in humans.

Intermittent fasting works by altering the body's circadian rhythm through a natural process called "autophagy," which is Greek for "self-eating." During fasting, your body is able to break down and clear out old proteins and cells. This is a natural procedure that aids to maintain optimal health and vitality. During autophagy, your body metabolizes fat instead of glucose for energy. This means that while you may still be eating the same number of calories each day, you are only losing fat instead of muscle or other lean tissue.

Fasting can improve your health in a number of ways:

- Intermittent fasting can benefit people with diabetes by helping them to better manage their blood sugar levels 24 hours after eating. Intermittent fasting can improve heart health by lowering triglyceride levels and improving "good" cholesterol. It also increases HDL, or "good," cholesterol, and lowers the number of LDL particles, which are considered the "bad" cholesterol.

- Intermittent fasting can help reduce body weight and body fat while maintaining lean muscle mass. This means you can lose more weight while improving your body composition. Not only will you look better, but you'll feel better too!

- Intermittent fasting may reduce symptoms of neurodegenerative diseases such as Alzheimer's disease and multiple sclerosis by decreasing inflammatory markers associated with these diseases. It may also normalize insulin production in those with Type II diabetes.

Origin of Intermittent Fasting

Intermittent fasting is not a new concept. It's been around for thousands of years and has seen a resurgence in popularity in recent years, particularly among bodybuilders and athletes.

The first known proponent of fasting was Hippocrates over 2,000 years ago. He believed that it was necessary to rid the body of all external factors in order to heal itself. He fasted his patients for long periods of time before prescribing medications and treatments. Research has since demonstrated that intermittent fasting can have many health benefits. The modern approaches are based on the 5:2 diet that was popularized by Michael Mosely's book, The Fast Diet: Lose Weight and Stay Healthy by Fasting Two Days a Week (2013).

Women Over 50

Women who have newly experienced menopause and are still in the process of adjusting to lower levels of estrogen may experience problems with intermittent fasting, including more acute signs of PMS. Women are generally more sensitive to dietary changes than men. Changes that they make quickly can bring on unexpected symptoms, both physical and emotional.

The main thing is that intermittent fasting is an instrument that can be used to improve health and to help manage disease. As with any other nutritional or dietary change, you should always consult your physician first. If you have been diagnosed with an eating disorder or other condition that requires nutritional counseling, working one-on-one with an experienced dietitian who is knowledgeable in this area can be extremely helpful.

This book will offer you all the necessary information on intermittent fasting and will give you a clear perspective of the practice and how it can help you in your quest for a healthier and long life.

We wish you all the best. Let us begin your journey?

Chapter 1: What is Intermittent Fasting?

First, let's get a little bit of background information on how and why people even think to use this method. Some people believe that eating less or fasting intermittently helps them lose weight easier by reducing their "calorie intake while maintaining nutrient density."

Others feel that intermittent fasting can help them stay healthier by reducing the amount of insulin, which is a hormone that allows you to carry glucose from your blood to the cells. Lastly, many people believe it's just a great way to improve their overall health and well-being. So how does all of this work?

Well, when eating meals or doing intermittent fasting, we are usually in what is called a "fed state" because the food you eat is providing glucose or sugar for your body to use. When you're in a fed state, you are stimulating the production of insulin, which is the hormone that enables you to carry glucose from your blood to the cells.

Intermittent fasting inhibits insulin secretion and also inhibits your body's ability to store fat. This is because when we eat, insulin actually blocks lipolysis (the process via which body fat is broken down into free fatty acids), so it allows your body to absorb excess sugar from your bloodstream.

After a period of not eating, however, insulin and blood sugar levels drop. This creates an "anabolic" environment for building muscle and losing body fat. During fasting, lipolysis is increased because the concentration of fatty acids in the bloodstream increases. What does this mean?

It means that fat cells break down into smaller fatty acids which are then released into the bloodstream to be used by the muscles as energy! So, what does this all mean? It essentially means that you can create an anabolic state for building muscle and losing body fat while fasting by having your glucose level drop below a certain threshold (usually around 70).

There are a few different ways to go about this, but the most common is called the 16/8 method. With this method, you would fast for 16 hours of the day and then eat for 8 hours. So, if you get up at 7 in the morning, you could not eat again until later that night at 9 PM.

Another way to do it is 8/16 or 12/12. The difference between these two methods is when your daily fast begins and ends. For those of you who are interested in this, I would highly recommend trying the 16/8 method and seeing what happens.

The reason for this is that it's more effective for fat loss and muscle gain than the other two methods. However, if you really prefer the 12/12 or 8/16 method, then do that instead. I just don't recommend trying all three methods at once because your results won't be as clear when you're not sticking to one method consistently.

Intermittent Fasting for Women Over 50

Intermittent fasting can help improve your health and your body composition, but the key is to not overdo it. It will be fine if you follow it for a couple of days a week—maybe even 4 times per week. But if you try to do it every single day, then that's how you can end up harming your body.

The first few days are going to be tough. Really tough! But you have to push through and I promise that when those first few days are done, you're going to feel amazing! So, start out slow and build up from there. You're going to be so happy that you did!

There are a few important rules to remember when fasting:

- It's best to stop eating at least 3 hours before you go to bed. This is important for a few reasons. First, while you sleep, your body is busy burning fat. You don't want to slow down that process by eating just before bedtime. Second, while you sleep, your body uses its glycogen stores as an energy source and the last thing you want is for those stores to run too low (which can cause muscle wasting).

- Don't exercise too late in the day. You can go on a walk in the morning or go to the gym in the afternoon, but don't do anything too strenuous later on in the day.

- Don't eat too close to bedtime. I know that you probably want to pack in as many calories as possible, but that isn't going to help you reach your goals…and if you fall asleep after eating a big meal, then your body will be less likely to use your fat stores as an energy source.

- Don't confuse skipping meals with intermittent fasting. Skipping meals usually leads to binge eating later on. If there is an event or something that you need to eat a little extra, then by all means do so. Just don't make a habit of it.

- Don't push your body too hard. If you're lifting weights in the morning, then go really easy on yourself for the rest of the day.

Chapter 2:   How Intermittent Fasting Works and the Science Behind It

Weight loss has emerged as a billion-dollar industry. It had a market valuation of over 70 billion last year. This is for an industry that didn't even exist a few decades back. The world didn't recognize obesity as a mainstream problem a century ago. Back then, malnutrition was a real problem. However, the circumstances have changed.

Today, obesity is a problem affecting more than 1.9 billion people all over the globe. However, have you ever wondered the reason most people fail to lose weight?

Weight loss is such a big problem because people don't address the correct issue.

Calories Are Not the Cause of Weight Gain

A very big misconception people have in their minds is that a few extra calories are the sole reason for their weight gain. They are wrong. Period.

Burning stored body fat is a much more complex process than you think. Until you don't understand the process, you will keep losing weight and burning body fat.

But, before that, you will have to understand that fat is important for the body and it fights tooth and nail to conserve this fat.

The Importance of Fat for the Body

Have you ever wondered the reason it is so difficult to burn body fat? It is so difficult because the body values this fat highly, and it tries everything to protect it.

Our body keeps collecting energy from almost every meal that we have and stores it as fat. It protects this fat aggressively because it knows that in a condition of complete energy cut-off, only this fat can help the body survive for the longest.

This is one reason your body won't start burning fat at the first instant of lower energy intake.

However, this is not the only reason your body doesn't begin burning fat immediately. There are two more reasons.

Important Factors for Burning Fat

To burn fat, only the energy deficit is not enough ground. Two more things will be required to burn fat. The first is readiness, and the second is the mode.

Let us understand both in detail:

Lack of Readiness—Insulin Resistance

Besides being the facilitator of glucose absorption, insulin is also the key fat-storage hormone. Whatever glucose is left in the bloodstream after the absorption of the cells, insulin stores it in the muscles, liver, and fat tissues.

The glucose in the bloodstream keeps the blood sugar levels high, which can be dangerous for the functioning of the vital organs. It can also affect crucial functions like blood pressure and elasticity of the muscles. High blood sugar content can harden the vessels, and they'll become prone to damage. That's the reason it is the job of insulin to lower the blood sugar levels rapidly.

This can be done fastest through absorption by the cells.

However, whatever glucose is left in the bloodstream, insulin starts storing it as glycogen in the muscles. But the muscles can't store a lot of it. As soon as the muscle glycogen stores are full, insulin starts storing glucose as glycogen in the liver.

The liver can store a substantial amount of energy. Your body can run only on the glycogen stored in the liver for almost 36 hours.

However, the glycogen stores of the liver keep filling up regularly, and hence insulin will not get to store a lot there.

The last place to store all the excess glucose is in the adipose tissues. A lot of fat can be stored as subcutaneous fat under your belly, thighs, and hips.

The Detrimental Impact of Insulin Resistance

As you know, insulin is a very important hormone, and it performs several crucial functions. Two key functions are facilitating glucose absorption by the cells and fat storage.

When your cells become insulin resistant, both these functions get affected.

First of all, cells respond slowly to the insulin signals, and hence your blood sugar levels remain high for longer than required. Due to this, the pancreas starts pumping more insulin as it wants the blood sugar levels to go down. However, more insulin is not solving the problem. More insulin means more exposure to the cells which are already battling overexposure. This escalates the problem further. This means that the cells wouldn't be in a condition to accept glucose readily, and the blood sugar levels would remain high. To solve this problem, insulin has no other option than to convert glucose into fat rapidly.

Now, insulin is the key fat-storage hormone. As long as there is a high insulin presence in your bloodstream, your body would remain in a fat-storage mode.

Once released by the pancreas, it takes anywhere between 8-12 hours for the insulin levels to go down. Because your body is battling insulin resistance, the insulin levels would be abnormally high because the pancreas keeps pumping more and more insulin.

This also means that your body would remain in a fat storage mode as the insulin levels are unlikely to go down in your body. From your last meal to the next meal, it takes anywhere between 8-12 hours for your insulin levels to go down. If you consume anything between this period, your insulin levels would again shoot up, and your body would stop burning any kind of fat.

Most of us never get that kind of a gap between our meals due to our erratic eating habits. This is one of the main reasons your body is unlikely to get into a fat-burning mode in normal conditions.

Our erratic eating habit at short intervals is one of the main culprits of insulin resistance and obesity. You must keep in mind that as long as your body is insulin resistant, it will struggle with fat burning.

Ketosis—The Fat Burning Mode

Another important reason for failing to burn fat is the wrong fuel mode.

Our body can run on two fuel types:

- The glucose fuels
- The fat fuels

You get glucose from the carbs and protein that you consume in your meals. The fat comes from the fat in the meat, fatty fruits, egg yolk, fatty fish, oils, etc.

Your body can easily run on both types of fuel. However, it can't run on both at the same time. When we are trying to lose weight with the calorie-restriction method or low-calorie diets, we are effectively trying to do just that. We lower the calorie and expect the body to burn fat and glucose at the same time.

This is not going to happen, and it never does. This is the reason most people never burn any real fat despite their best efforts.

The process of burning fat is called ketosis. In this process, your body switches from glucose fuel to fat fuel. Once the body has made the switch, and it is only getting fat fuel to burn, it will easily start burning the body fat as fuel.

However, for this to take place, you will have to stop the intake of glucose fuel. This means that you will have to stop the intake of carbs and would also have to manage your protein intake strictly as excess protein would also get converted into glucose, ultimately through the process of glucogenesis.

Burning Fat in Reality

If you want to burn fat, you will have to ensure no excess insulin is floating in your bloodstream. You will have to keep in mind that no matter what, as long as there is insulin in your bloodstream, your body wouldn't start burning fat as it would remain in a fat storage mode.

This is where intermittent fasting is of special use.

Intermittent fasting is the process of creating prolonged gaps between your meals. With the help of intermittent fasting, you will be able to create longer gaps so that the insulin levels can go down for very long. In such circumstances, your body would be able to burn fat for energy.

Intermittent fasting is also the best way to lower insulin resistance, and hence you can also expect your cells to become more sensitive to insulin signals. This means that there will be less insulin in your bloodstream if your cells respond well to the insulin signals.

Intermittent fasting also creates long gaps of glucose absence. Glucose is a short-lived form of energy. This means that your cells can use glucose rapidly. It provides instant energy, but it doesn't last very long. Hence, if you are more insulin sensitive, your cells would absorb glucose rapidly and use it up fast.

If you consume food again after a short interval, your body will start facing energy shortage. In the complete absence of glucose, your body can also begin ketosis, in which it starts breaking fats to convert them into ketones that can be used as energy.

A fat-rich diet like a ketogenic diet, also called the keto diet, will expedite the process.

The fat you consume in your diet doesn't get processed in the same way as glucose. It is broken down in the intestines with the help of bile juices released by the gallbladder.

The bile juices help in breaking the fat into smaller parts, and these are then metabolized in the liver. However, unlike glucose, you don't need insulin to facilitate the absorption of the ketones by the cells. To facilitate the absorption of ketones, the alpha cells in the pancreas releases glucagon. Hence, there is no insulin response at all in your body. This means that your body will be capable of burning the body fat right away if there is any significant need for energy like heavy exercise.

Therefore, it is with the help of intermittent fasting and a keto diet that you can easily achieve fat-burning much faster and more effectively than any other process.

It is one of the most reliable ways to lose weight rapidly.

You would lose a significant amount of your actual body fat without following a punishing diet or calorie-restriction program. Intermittent fasting is the most scientific way to lose significant weight without compromising your health.

Hormonal Health of Women—The Most Ignored Factor in Weight Loss

One of the most dangerous things that women do while trying to lose weight is that they ignore the importance of their hormonal health.

One of the most significant differences between men and women is the way their bodies treat food. The body of a man doesn't attach too much significance to food. For men, food is just a way to survive. This is in stark contrast to the way the body of a woman treats food.

For women, food means much more than simple survival; it is connected to their hormonal balance. Since the time a girl hits puberty to the time she reaches menopause, her body is physically always in a readiness mode to bear a child. Bearing a child is a big responsibility. A child in the womb is a big drain on the energy sources in a woman's body. Once a woman conceives a child, her body tries its best to provide nutrition to the child. This was always not possible through conventional mediums in the past.

In the past, women sometimes got food and, most of the time, they didn't. This can make the survival of the child in the womb difficult. To solve this problem, nature has devised the plan of energy storage inside the body to help the child survive.

This is why women have a comparatively higher body fat ratio than men, and they are also more likely to gain fat rapidly. It is not a weakness they have, but a brilliant plan devised by nature to help the coming generations survive.

Food and Female Hormones Are Connected

The hormones in the body are chemical messengers that help in passing on vital information to the brain. Hormones regulate several crucial functions. If you look closely, the life of a woman is completely dominated by these hormones.

The thyroid and pituitary are two very important glands that secrete most of the hormones. They also regulate the behavior of a woman. These glands are also present in men but don't have that profound impact on them simply because they are not going to bear a child.

Women feel a very strong connection with food, and that's why emotional eating, impulsive eating, celebration eating, and all other forms of eating have such strong meanings for women.

For women, food is a part of emotional security as it also helps in the regulation and balancing of certain hormones.

Impact of Calories—Restrictive Diets of Hormonal Balance

Calorie-restrictive diets can harm the hormonal balance in women. It can fill them with a sense of insecurity, void, and unhappiness. Scientific experiments on mice have shown that prolonged calorie-restriction can also lead to the shrinking of female reproductive organs, and they may also lose their ability to reproduce effectively.

Strict diets can also cause irregular periods, and they may also face problems in conception. Women on calorie-restrictive diets can also experience strong and sudden mood swings, and they may also become more temperamental. Anger, frustration, irritation, hopelessness, temptation, and cravings are some of the strong feelings experienced by women on calorie-restrictive diets.

Hormonal Balance is Important

It is very important to understand that hormonal balance is very important. Without the hormonal balance, the overall health of a woman will always remain compromised. This is the problem most women keep facing all their lives.

In the pursuit of weight loss and a slender body, women compromise on their hormonal health and end up paying for problems like PCOS, thyroid, metabolic disorders, and other reproductive issues.

Intermittent Fasting—A Reliable Way to Lose Weight Without Compromising Hormonal Health

Intermittent fasting is a safe way to lose weight as it doesn't force you to compromise your hormonal health. Intermittent fasting doesn't make you starve for food or limit your calorie intake specifically.

It is a process that allows you to eat reasonably. There are no calorie restrictions. You can eat whatever you feel like as long as you maintain adequate control over quantity.

This eliminates cravings, temptations, and obsessiveness regarding certain food items, and hence your hormones remain in control.

Intermittent fasting is not about what to eat but when to eat. The most important thing in intermittent fasting is to observe abstinence from food for a certain number of hours every day. This period can be efficiently timed to be your sleep time, and hence severe hunger pangs and cravings can easily be avoided.

Chapter 3: Myths About Intermittent Fasting

The next step would be to rid our minds of certain myths that people have initiated about intermittent fasting over the years. One credible characteristic of the human mouth and hands is their ability to talk and write critically. People would always have a different view and not flow in synergy with what is brought to the table irrespective of how prospect-filled it may appear. Certain myths have come up over the years about the concept of intermittent fasting and it would only be fair to have me address this in this book. Here are a few:

Intermittent Fasting Is a Road to Starvation

A little enlightenment on this would be in order. Starvation is a condition where someone suffers severely due to a lack of food. It is wrong to think that not eating for 24-48 hours starves the body. Research has inadvertently shown that for the body to get started and experience a reduction in metabolic rate, an individual has to not eat for over 60 hours. That is almost three days. As individuals, tight work schedules prevent us from eating for a more significant part of the day and even though we expend a lot of energy doing our work, we still do not break down.

The Burden of Hunger

Some others say that you will feel hungry all day long while doing intermittent fasting. The human body is very adaptive. That is why impoverished or poor individuals can stay for almost a day without food. They are healthy and working tirelessly. From the second week of intermittent fasting, hunger gets low; your body adjusts to your new routine. Just as your body adjusts when saddled with more energy-consuming activities. Here's another thing; most times we are most likely to feel hungry easily when we are in an idle state (doing nothing). Something else you could do is to keep yourself busy all the while during your fasting periods. Getting busy takes our minds away from a lot of things including food, we're fully focused on what we have at hand.

Eating Frequently Boosts Your Metabolism

Now, it is another myth generally acknowledged by many people that eating often boosts metabolism. We cannot deny that calories are expended in metabolic processes; this is very true. This is also seen in the digestion of food and is known as the Thermic Effect of Food. The body uses about 10% of your overall calorie intake to do this. On the other hand, now, here's where this myth is faulting. What matters is not how frequently you eat, but the number of calories you eat. Now, someone consuming six meals of about 500 calories is the same as consuming three meals containing a thousand calories. Therefore, this myth is wrong.

Dietary Glucose for the Brain

Here's another common misconception. Some people believe that if you do not eat carbs every once in a while, your brain will cease to function. The reason for this is that the brain uses glucose as its only source of fuel. On the other hand, this myth is faulted too because of the concept of gluconeogenesis. This is a process whereby the body synthesizes glucose from non-carbohydrate sources. During long fasts, such as this and low-carb dieting, your body can produce ketone bodies from dietary fats. These ketone bodies feed a part of the brain until it significantly reduces its glucose requirements.

Reduction in Muscle Mass

People have also concluded that intermittent fasting reduces body mass. Although this sometimes happens during fasting, any experiment hasn't proved that it happens more with intermittent fasting than other fast forms. Recent studies show a significant increase in muscle mass for individuals who consume all the calorie requirement in one big meal in a day. It is a predominant technique among bodybuilders, it maintains the muscles. It enhances a considerable amount of weight loss with minimal reduction in muscle mass. This myth is flawed as much evidence proves that intermittent fasts have minimal effect on muscle mass.

Incessant Eating Ensures Good Health

People think that when they eat incessantly, they make good health. This is not entirely true. The body indeed requires nutrients and energy to thrive. Still, cellular repair processes are engaged during intermittent fast periods. This cellular repair process known as Autophagy uses dysfunctional and waste proteins for energy. It also prevents aging, cancer and Alzheimer's disease. Some studies have shown that snacking and eating regularly most times harm your body in different ways. For example, when you take a diet with many calories, you cause your liver to become fatty, making you more likely to get fatty liver disease.

Additionally, some research has come up to say that you put yourself in more danger of colorectal cancer if you eat often. Therefore, this further proves that intermittent fast has more health and metabolic benefits than you could imagine.

Skipping Breakfast Can Make You Fat

I also don't know how this myth came about or how it came to be believed. Well, that is how myths are. It is thought that skipping breakfast increases your meal cravings, thus making you consume more food. However, research has proven that skipping breakfast does not have any signs of individuals' weight gain or otherwise. Therefore, you must pay attention to your specific needs. Breakfast is a must for some people and some others can do without it.

Indiscipline Eating Habits on Work Days

Now, your engaging in intermittent fasting does not give you the leverage to be glutton and eat whatever enters your view. In as much as intermittent fasting helps burn up a lot of calories, replacing the burnt-up calories with even more significant amounts on fast-off days provides counter-productive results. It's like shooting yourself on the leg. You take away a piece of dirt and bring in a basket full. At all times, healthy eating habits should be maintained. Adequate and healthy calorie consumption should be checked and monitored. This is why it is mostly advised that you begin intermittent fasts with a dietician/doctor's assistance. Do not pull down your big house of cards with your own hands; self-discipline is a principal element that can help.

Intermittent Fasting Is Never Ending

Here's another myth; some people have themselves and others believe that once you begin an intermittent fast, you have to keep it going for life. Now to these sets of people, I would love to ask the straightforward question; "What was the purpose of the fast in the first place?" To burn up a lot of calories and mostly achieve weight loss, not so? Now, this eating plan being effective is seeing that the desired result has been achieved. Once the desired results have been seen, there is no need to continue with the exercise. All you need to do from then is watch what you eat, so you won't get excessive calories stored up again. Intermittent fasting helps you train your taste buds to loathe foods with a high percentage of calories; you don't have to struggle to abstain from them anymore after staying through to the intermittent fasting plan for you.

These myths do not clamp down the efficacy of the intermittent fasting method. Logically and ideally, intermittent fasting has more health and metabolic benefits than can be seen. Maybe they just choose to ignore the pros and focus on the cons. The benefits of Intermittent fasting, even over very short terms, cannot be over-emphasized. Fasting exposes the body to a lot of beneficial processes that bulky calories would not let it access. Gene expressions, metabolic waste removal processes, the formation of new neurons and cellular repair are some of these beneficial processes that go on in the body during fasting to mention, but just a few.

Chapter 4:   Benefits of Intermittent Fasting

Weight Loss

Intermittent Fasting switches from periods of eating to periods of fasting. If you fast, naturally, your calorie intake will reduce, and it also helps you maintain your weight loss. It also prevents you from indulging in mindless eating. Whenever you eat something, your body converts the food into glucose and fat. It uses this glucose immediately and stores the fat for later use. When you skip a few meals, your body starts to reach into its internal stores of fat to provide energy. Also, most of the fat that you lose is from the abdominal region. If you want a flat tummy, then this is the perfect diet for you.

Tackles Diabetes

Diabetes is a significant threat on its own. It is also a primary indicator of the increase in risk factors of various cardiovascular diseases like heart attacks and strokes. When the glucose level increases alarmingly in the bloodstream, and there isn't enough insulin to process this glucose, it causes diabetes. When your body resists insulin, it becomes difficult to regulate insulin levels in the body. Intermittent Fasting reduces insulin sensitivity and helps tackle diabetes.

Sleep

Lack of sleep is one of the main causes of obesity. When your body doesn't get enough sleep, the internal mechanism of burning fat suffers. Intermittent Fasting regulates your sleep cycle and, in turn, makes your body effectively burn fats. A good sleep cycle has different physiological benefits—it makes you feel energetic and elevates your overall mood.

Resistance to Illnesses

Intermittent Fasting helps in the growth and regeneration of cells. Did you know that the human body has an internal mechanism that helps repair damaged cells? Intermittent Fasting helps kickstart this mechanism. It improves the overall functioning of all the cells in the body. So, it is directly responsible for improving your body's natural defense mechanism by increasing its resistance to diseases and illnesses.

A Healthy Heart

Intermittent Fasting assists in weight loss, and weight loss improves your cardiovascular health. A buildup of plaque in blood vessels is known as atherosclerosis. This is the primary cause of various cardiovascular diseases. The endothelium is the thin lining of blood vessels, and any dysfunction in it results in atherosclerosis. Obesity is the primary problem that plagues humanity and is also the main reason for the increase of plaque deposits in the blood vessels. Stress and inflammation also increase the severity of this problem. Intermittent Fasting tackles the buildup of fat and helps tackle obesity. So, all you need to do is follow the simple protocols of Intermittent Fasting to improve your overall health.

A Healthy Gut

There are several millions of microorganisms present in your digestive system. These microorganisms help improve the overall functioning of your digestive system and are known as the gut microbiome. Intermittent Fasting enhances the health of these microbiomes and improves your digestive health. A healthy digestive system helps in better absorption of food and improves the functioning of your stomach.

Reduces Inflammation

Whenever your body feels there is an internal problem, its natural defense is inflammation. It doesn't mean that all forms of inflammation are desirable. Inflammation can cause several serious health conditions like arthritis, atherosclerosis, and other neurodegenerative disorders.
Any inflammation of this nature is known as chronic inflammation and is quite painful. Chronic inflammation can restrict your body's movements too. If you want to keep inflammation in check, then Intermittent Fasting will certainly come in handy.

Promotes Cell Repair

When you fast, the cells in your body start the process of waste removal. Waste removal means the breaking down of all dysfunctional cells and proteins and is known as autophagy. Autophagy offers protection against several degenerative diseases like Alzheimer's and cancer. You don't like accumulating garbage in your home, do you? Similarly, your body must not hold onto any unnecessary toxins. Autophagy is the body's way of getting rid of all things useless.

Higher Concentration and Brain Power

When subjected to food scarcity for a long time, mammals, including humans, will start to experience a decrease in their organ size. One of these organs is the brain. While some organs return to their original size over time, others may be impacted over the long term.

The brain handles the basic cognitive function of the body. In order to function properly and get the needed nutrients, it needs to return to its original size. However, if the brain becomes too foggy, getting the needed food nutrients will be pretty difficult, which might lead to malnutrition and even be fatal. However, during a shorter period of food scarcity, the brain becomes hyperactive in its search for food as a mechanism for survival.

Excessive availability of food and eating altogether makes us mentally dull. Reflect on a time when you were completely satisfied after a big meal. After eating a massive plate of food, you will likely go into a "food coma" and curl up and sleep, or maybe just watch your favorite TV show on Netflix rather than get the motivation to go achieve your goals. Without a doubt, satisfaction from food makes man naturally lose the drive to pursue his goals, which ultimately leads to dulling the brain. With this in mind, know that when you fast, your cognitive abilities are quickened. This improves your mental keenness, allowing you to achieve your health-related goals as opposed to excessively feeding.

It should be established here that there is no scientific research to support the notion that intermittent fasting alters mental alertness negatively. Fasting will not affect your cognitive function, such as moods, mental alertness, reaction time, intention, and sleep in any bad way. On the contrary, these things get boosted during fasting.

Fasting Promotes Autophagy and Protects Neurons

This is one of the many wonderful benefits of intermittent fasting, which many people should look forward to. Fasting is amazing in that it keeps the brain's cells from degeneration. This is because fasting prevents neural death.

Besides, fasting also triggers the process of autophagy in the brain—autophagy is the process in which the body gets rid of damaged body cells and brings out new ones. When the body is full of healthy, active, and improved cells, it is strong and well-equipped to combat any diseases that might want to attack.

With autophagy, the risk of viral infection, as well as duplication of intracellular parasites, reduces drastically. This dramatically reduces intracellular pathogens, such as cancer cells. Besides, the brain and other body tissue cells are protected from abnormal growth, inflammation, and toxicity.

Reduced Risk of Depression

With intermittent fasting, there is an increase in the levels of a neurotransmitter called "neurotrophic factor." When the body is deficient in this brain-derived factor, it contributes to significant issues such as depression and other mood disorders. Hence, intermittent fasting is really helpful in improving mental alertness and enhancing mood, which ultimately leads to a reduced tendency to develop these conditions.

There are a couple of metabolic features that get triggered when we fast that improve brain health. This explains why people who practice intermittent fasting do have lower levels of inflammation, low blood sugar levels, and reduced oxidative stress.

There are also indications that intermittent fasting can keep the brain protected against the risk of stroke.

Intermittent Fasting Fosters Immune Regulation

When you fast, part of the primary aim of the body is to keep the immune system healthy. This is why we encourage drinking a large quantity of water during the period of the intermittent fast, and afterward as well. Water can be spiced up with other detox agents that remove toxins from the digestive system and reduces the number of unhealthy gut microbes. Have in mind that the number of gut microbes present in the gastrointestinal tract is directly related to the immune system's function. Intermittent fasting determines the number of inflammatory cytokines that the body has. Hence, it helps regulate the body's overall immune system. In the body, we have two significant cytokines that cause inflammation in the body: Interleukin-6 and Tumor Necrosis Factor Alpha. Fasting suppresses the release of these inflammatory pro-inflammatory cytokines.

Intermittent Fasting Reduces the Risk of Chronic Disease

People living with chronic autoimmune diseases like Crohn's disease, colitis, rheumatoid arthritis, and systemic lupus will definitely see remarkable improvement with intermittent fasting. The idea is simple. Fasting reduces the rate of an extreme inflammatory process in the bodies of these persons. With this, they have an ideal immune function.

For instance, cancer cells have between ten and seventy extra insulin receptors in contrast to healthy body cells. This happens as a result of the breakdown of sugar for fuel. With intermittent fasting, cancer cells are starved of sugar intake. This conditions the cells for damage through free radicals.

Improves Genetic Repair Mechanisms

The tendency of the body to live longer increases when it does not get enough food. This is because, with intermittent fasting, there is repair and regeneration of cells that come about via a repair mechanism in the body. This is understandable, as the energy required for cell repair is lesser when compared to what is necessary for cell creation or division.

Hence, during the period of intermittent fasting, cell division, and creation in the body becomes reduced. This is a necessary process, vital especially for the healing of malignant cells, which thrive as a result of abnormal cell division.

In the body, the human growth hormone (HGH) takes care of the process of cell repair. It is a human growth hormone that brings out changes in metabolism that cause tissue repair and fat burning. Thus, when we fast, the body can concentrate more on repairing body tissues with amino acids and enzymes. This restores tissue collagen and also triggers an improvement in bones, ligaments, tendons, and general muscle function in the body.

Reduce the Likelihood of Developing Cancer

Lastly, studies have found that intermittent fasting can reduce your likelihood of developing cancer and help make treatment more successful. As you are aware, intermittent fasting can help treat oxidative stress and cellular damage, both of which cause cancer. By reducing this damage, you can thereby reduce your risk of developing cancer in the future.

But that is not all. While human studies still need to be conducted, a study on mice found that when practicing short-term fasting, chemotherapy treatment becomes more successful in targeting and treating both breast cancer and skin cancer. Not only did the chemotherapy itself become more effective, but the mice' immune systems also were better able to fight off the cancerous cells and growths, which is essential as chemotherapy is well-known for reducing a person's immune system drastically.

Chapter 5:   Downsides and Possible Risks of Intermittent Fasting

Moving to longer fasts is a decision that must be taken very carefully.

Here are possible risks and downsides of Intermittent Fasting:

The Hormonal Balance

The first and foremost consideration is hormonal balance. Women have a very unique system. Hormones play a very crucial role in their body and have a very strong attachment to their energy needs. While the body of a woman likes to store excess fat as compared to men, the impact of food security is also psychological. These are some reasons women must be very careful while fasting at a young age.

Fasts longer than 14 hours are not suggested for women in their reproductive age. This is irrespective of their desire to have more kids or not. In the childbearing age or before the age a woman reaches menopause, the body is releasing a lot of hormones that are highly sensitive to insulin signals. Fasting for unnecessarily long periods can be very harmful.

However, as you reach menopause, fasting becomes more feasible. Your hormonal balance stops reacting so sharply to hunger response and hence you are in a better position to keep for longer periods. But this doesn't give you a permit to be reckless in your fasting routine. Fasting must always be carried out in a disciplined manner as it is a big change for your whole body. You must always move up your fasting hours swiftly and ensure that your body is well adjusted to the routine. If even after a few days of being on a routine you don't feel well adjusted, then probably that fasting routine is not your cup of tea.

Necessity

Most women feel the desire to keep longer fasts because they want to lose fat rapidly. There are women with other health conditions who want to go on longer fasts for rapid relief but the ratio of women trying to lose weight quickly with longer fasts is disproportionate. However, what they don't try to understand is that the weight loss with most fasting schedules is almost similar. It doesn't matter whether you are keeping 14-hours fasts or 16-hours fasts, the weight loss would be very similar. The major impact of the fast duration would be on other health conditions like insulin resistance, HGH production, blood pressure regulation, etc.

The impact of the duration of the fast on weight loss is very low and hence you do not need to take the risk of upsetting your hormonal balance for such a minuscule gain. If you keep following the intermittent fasting routine, to which you are well adjusted, you will be able to lose weight much faster and sustain it better.

Nutrient Deficiency

A big consideration with longer fasting is nutrient deficiency. It is always very important for women to ensure that they are getting the required nutrition. Nutrient deficiency in women is a very common problem.

Fasting can create a bit of a problem in this area as your usual food intake goes down. If you extend your fasting hours too much, you will be putting your nutrition at risk. You might not get the required nutrition and fall prey to other health issues. Therefore, you must get the required nutrition and not take the risk of unusually longer fasts.

Chapter 6:   Various Types of Intermittent Fasting

16/8 Method

This is just about the most popular fasting methods since it's so schedule-based, meaning there are no surprises. This will give you the freedom to control when you eat, based on your everyday life. Sixteen is the number of hours you're likely to be fasting, which may also be lowered to twelve or perhaps fourteen hours if that better fits into your life. Then, you're eating period is going to be between eight and ten hours every day. This might seem daunting, but it just means that you are skipping an entire meal. Many people choose to begin their fast around 7 or 8 p.m. and then not eating until 11 or noon the next day, which means they fast for the recommended 16 hours. Of course, it isn't as bad as it sounds, since they are sleeping during this time, so what it comes down to is eating dinner and then not eating again until the next day around lunch, so you are just skipping breakfast.

You will be doing it every day, so finding the hours that work for you is important. If you work the third shift, then switching you're eating period around to fit into your schedule is important. If you find yourself being run down and sluggish, tweak your fasting hours until you find a healthy balance. Granted, there will be some adjustment, because, chances are your body is not accustomed to skipping entire meals. However, this should go away after a couple of weeks, and if it doesn't then try starting your fasting period earlier in the day allowing you to eat earlier the next, or alter it however you need to feel healthy and happy.

Lean-Gains Method (14:10)

The lean-gains method has several different incarnations on the web, but its fame comes from the fact that it helps shed fat while building it into muscle almost immediately. Through the lean-gains method, you'll find yourself able to change all that fat into muscle through a rigorous practice of fasting, eating right, and exercising.

Through this method, you fast anywhere from 14 to 16 hours and spend the remaining 10 or 8 hours each day engaged in eating and exercising. As opposed to the crescendo, this method features daily fasting and eating, rather than alternated days of eating versus not. Therefore, you don't have to be quite cautious about extending the physical effort to exercise on the days you are fasting because those days when you're fasting are every day!

For the lean-gaining method, start fasting only for 14 hours and work it up to 16 if you feel comfortable with it, but never forget to drink enough water and be careful about spending too much energy on exercise! Remember that you want to grow in health and potential through intermittent fasting. You'll certainly not want to lose any of that growth by forcing the process along.

20:4 Method

Stepping things up a notch from the 14:10 and 16:8 methods, the 20:4 method is a tough one to master, for it is rather unforgiving. People talk about this method of intermittent fasting as intense and highly restrictive. Still, they also say that the effects of living this method are almost unparalleled with all other tactics.

For the 20:4 method, you'll fast for 20 hours each day and squeeze all your meals, all your eating, and all your snacking into 4 hours. People who attempt 20:4 normally have two smaller meals or just one large meal and a few snacks during their 4-hour window to eat, and it is up to the individual which four hours of the day they devote to eating.

The trick for this method is to make sure you're not overeating or bingeing during those 4-hour windows to eat. It is all-too-easy to get hungry during the 20-hour fast and have that feeling then propel you into intense and unrealistic hunger or meal sizes after the fast period is over. Be careful if you try this method. If you're new to intermittent fasting, work your way up to this one gradually, and if you're working your way up already, only make the shift to 20:4 when you know you're ready. It would surely be disappointing if all your progress with intermittent fasting got hijacked by one poorly thought-out goal with the 20:4 method.

Meal Skipping

Meal skipping is an extremely flexible form of intermittent fasting that can provide all of the benefits of intermittent fasting but with less strict scheduling. If you are not someone who has a typical schedule or feels like a stricter variation of the intermittent fasting diet will serve you, meal skipping is a viable alternative.

Many people who choose to use meal skipping find it a great way to listen to their bodies and follow their basic instincts. If they are not hungry, they simply don't eat that meal. Instead, they wait for the next one. Meal skipping can also help people who have time constraints and who may not always be able to get in a certain meal of the day.

It is important to realize that with meal skipping, you may not always be maintaining a 10-16-hour window of fasting. As a result, you may not get every benefit that comes from other fasting diets. However, this may be a great solution for people who want an intermittent fasting diet that feels more natural. It may also be a great idea for those looking to begin listening to their bodies more so that they can adjust to a more intense variation of the diet with greater ease. It can be a great transitional diet for you if you are not ready to jump into one of the other fasting diets just yet.

Warrior Diet Fasting

The most extreme form of intermittent fasting is known as the Warrior Diet. This intermittent fasting cycle follows a 20-hour fasting window with a short 4-hour eating window. During that eating window, individuals are supposed to only consume raw fruits and vegetables. They can also eat one large meal. Typically, the eating window occurs at night time so people can snack throughout the evening, have a large meal, and then resume fasting.

Because of the length of fasting taking place during the Warrior Diet, people should also consume a fairly hearty level of healthy fats. Doing so will give the body something to consume during the fast to produce energy with. A small amount of carbohydrates can also be incorporated to support energy levels, too.

People who eat the Warrior Diet tend to believe that humans are natural nocturnal eaters and that we are not meant to eat throughout the day. The belief is that eating this way follows our natural circadian rhythms, allowing our body to work optimally.

The only people who should consider doing the Warrior Diet are those who have already had success with other forms of intermittent fasting and who are used to it. Attempting to jump straight into the Warrior Diet can have serious repercussions for anyone who is not used to intermittent fasting. Even still, those who are used to it may find this particular style too extreme for them to maintain.

Eat-Stop-Eat (24 Hour) Method

This method of fasting is incredibly similar to the crescendo method. The only discernable difference is that there's no anticipation of increasing into a more intense fasting pattern with time. For the eat-stop-eat method, you decide which days you want to take off from eating, and then you run with it until you've lost that weight and then you keep running with the lifestyle for good because you won't be able to imagine life without it.

The eat-stop-eat method involves one to two days a week being 100% oriented towards fasting, with the other five to six days concerning "business as normal." The one or two days spent fasting are then full 24-hour days spent without eating anything at all. These days, of course, water and coffee are still fine to drink, but no food items can be consumed whatsoever. Exercise is also frowned upon on those fasting days, but see what your body can handle before you decide how that should all work out. Some people might start thinking they're using the crescendo method but end up sticking with eat-stop-eat.

Alternate-Day Method

The alternate-day method is admittedly a little confusing, but the reason it could be so confusing could come, in part, from how much wiggle room it provides for the practitioner. This method is great for people who don't have a consistent schedule or any sense of one, it is incredibly forgiving for those who don't quite have everything together for themselves yet.

When it comes down to it, alternate-day intermittent fasting is really up to you. You should try to fast every other day, but it doesn't have to be that precise. Similarly, with the crescendo method, as long as you fast two to three days a week, with a break day or two in between each fasting day, you're set! Then, you'll want to eat normally for three or four days out of each week, and when you encounter a fasting day, you don't even need to completely fast!

Alternate-day fasting is a solid place to start from, especially if you work a varying schedule or still have yet to get used to a consistent one. If you want to make things more intense from this starting point, the alternate-day method can easily become the eat-stop-eat method, the crescendo method, or the 5:2 method. Essentially, this method is a great place to begin

12:12 Method

As another of the more natural ways of intermittent fasting, the 12:12 approach is well-suited to beginning practitioners. Many people live out the 12:12 method without any forethought simply because of their sleeping and eating schedule, but turning the 12:12 into a conscious practice can have just as many positive effects on your life as the more drastic 20:4 method claims.

According to a study conducted in the University of Alabama, for this method in particular, you fast for 12 hours and then enter a 12-hour eating window. It's not difficult whatsoever to get three small meals and several snacks, or two big meals and a snack into your day with this method. With the 12:12, the standard meal timing works just fine.

Ultimately, this method is a great one to start from, for a lot of variation can be built into this scheduling when you're ready to make things more interesting. Effortlessly and without much effort, 12:12 can become 14:10 or even 16:8, and in seemingly no time, you can find yourself trying alternate-day or crescendo methods, too. Start with what's normal for you, and this method might be exactly that!

5:2 Method

This is another popular way to fast, because there is no true fasting involved, but instead, a strict and drastic calorie reduction for two days each week. So, for five days a week, you will eat your normal 1,600 to 2,000 calories and exercise like normal. On two non-consecutive days a week, you will restrict your caloric intake to between 500 and 600 calories. When doing this, pay close attention to the number of calories in beverages as well, many people make the mistake of only counting calories in what they eat. Remember, that beverages contain calories too, especially if you are drinking things from coffee shops, as these tend to have high amounts of sugar.

Crescendo Method

This is usually an introduction to fasting, it is how many people begin their fasting journey. This is a less-intense form of intermittent fasting and is a great way for you to see how it works to ease your fears and become familiarized with a fasting schedule. This method involves normally 4 or 5 days a week and then restricting you're eating period to between 8 or 10 hours for two or three non-consecutive days. Very similar to the 16/8 method, but instead of doing it every day, you only do it a couple of days each week. These are the safest ways for women to fast because they do not upset the body's hormonal balance. Intermittent fasting not done properly can trick the body into going into what is known as starvation mode. This happens when the body thinks it needs to hold onto fat longer because it doesn't know when it will have a chance to consume food for fuel again. This can lead to burning muscle for fuel and upsetting the hormonal balance, leading to even more issues. However, intermittent fasting done properly can be safe and incredibly beneficial.
Intermittent fasting helps you lose weight, but it also improves mental clarity and simplifies your life in a way that diets do not. Consider the length of time spent worrying about or perhaps eating food, and then imagine what other things you can be doing if this weren't the case. This's one of the main benefits of intermittent fasting, you will find no surprises and can take total control of when you eat.

Chapter 7: Tips and Tricks to Start Intermittent Fasting

There are a few things you have to remember whether you need to shed pounds with intermittent fasting, here below the main four:

- Food quality: The food you eat is still important. Try to eat whole and simply seasoned foods.
- Calories: Calories, despite everything still count. Try to eat "typically" during the eating periods and not to make up for the calories you missed by fasting.
- Consistency: Just like any other weight-loss strategy, you have to stick with it for the long term if you want it to work.
- Patience: It will take as much time as is needed to get used to an intermittent fasting lifestyle. Try to be consistent with your meal calendar, and it will get simpler.

The greater part of the famous intermittent fasting methods also suggests food quality. This is significant in case you need to lose body fat while keeping muscle.

In the beginning, calorie counting is commonly not required with intermittent fasting. If your weight loss slows down, then calorie counting can be a useful practice.

With intermittent fasting, you, despite everything, need to eat healthily and keep up a calorie shortage if you need to get in shape.

Defining Specific Measurable Goals

Rather than setting a general goal like "getting fitter," be more specific, focus on basic, feasible objectives that should be possible week by week, like:

- Taking a walk three days per week
- Drink 64 ounces of water per day, every day, this week
- Skip one meal this week

Self-Reward When Reaching Small Targets

Set yourself up for progress by utilizing a prize framework. For example:

- After shedding fifteen pounds, get yourself some new clothes.
- If you meet all your monthly goals, treat yourself to a massage.

The cash spared by skipping a meal (or two) can pay for your prize! Things that can motivate us are different for every one of us, so make sure to find out what might work best for you, and you will stay focused on reaching all of your goals.

Keeping a Journal

This is quite a game-changer. If you have a very strong willpower and you are used to doing medium to long term plans and sticking to them, you probably won't need to keep a journal, if not for the pleasure to do it, and unless this already is one of the tools behind your willpower.

Most of us, though, are not like this. The ability to stick to a plan (dietary or of any other nature) is seldom a talent. More often than you think, there are tools and practices involved. When it comes to diets, especially, but not only, if the aim is to lose weight, the number one cause of quitting is the lack of immediate and measurable results. Or at least this is the reason the quitter, in all honesty, gives. But is it really about this? Well, not exactly. Most of the time, it is not that one does not have results, it is that they have in mind the big final goal, therefore they can't appreciate the small ones during the journey.

If your final goal is to save 10.000 dollars, you won't get excited about your first 10 dollars saved. If your final goal is to lift 200 pounds, you won't get excited about your first 20 pounds lifted. If your final goal is to shed 20 pounds, you won't get excited about your first 10 ounces shed. But the truth is, to save 10.000 dollars, to lift 200 pounds, to shed 20 pounds, you have to start saving 10, lifting 20, shedding just your first ten ounces.

This is the main use of journaling: keeping track day-by-day of the small victories to celebrate and the small struggles to fight, being able to have everything under control and to love and appreciate the journey, until you won't need to keep track anymore and either will quit doing it, or will keep on just for the pleasure of it.

Once you know what to keep track of, it is very easy, and pleasant, to do it. Not only it is the chance to track your progress, but it also is something that gives you a moment that is all yours, where you can, in some way, talk to yourself.

I usually suggest setting a "three-month challenge" because this is, give or take, the period of time in which you may see yourself as a "beginner" of intermittent fasting. Usually, after three months you are in the zone, you just acquired the intermittent fasting lifestyle as your own and you don't need to journal about it anymore (of course you can, some people do it, but it becomes more of a pleasure than a tool).

6 Ways to Make a Fast Diet Effective

Know Your Weight, BMI and Waist Size from the Start

As mentioned earlier, waist measurement is an essential and straightforward measure of internal fat and a strong predictor of future health. People with intermittent fasting quickly lose those dangerous and unattractive centimeters. The BMI is the square of the weight (in kilograms) divided by the height (in meters). It looks ugly and may sound abstract, but it is a widely-used tool to find a way to healthy weight loss. The BMI values do not take into account your body type, age, or ethnicity. You should, therefore, consider yourself informed. However, this is useful when you need a number.

Weigh yourself regularly. After the first phases, once a week is enough. If you want the numbers to drop, the morning after fasting is your best bet. Researchers at the University of Illinois noted: "Weighing can vary significantly from food to fasting days. This weight deviation is probably due to the extra weight of food in the digestive tract."

It is not a daily change in fat mass. Future solutions may require solutions that try averaging the weight measurements on consecutive feeding and fasting days to determine weight more accurately. There are 28 tasks. If you are a person who likes structure and clarity, you may want to track your progress. Think about your goals. When and where do you want to go? Be realistic: rapid weight loss is not recommended. Please take your time. Make a plan. Write it down.

Many people recommend keeping a diet journal. Add your experience next to the number. Note the three good things that happen every day. It is a message of happiness that can be referenced over time.

Find a Fasting Friend

You need very few accessories to be successful, but a supportive friend can be one of them. Once you are on the fast diet, tell people about it; you may find that they join you, and you will build a network of shared experiences. As the plan appeals to both men and women, couples report that doing it together is more comfortable. This way, you get mutual support, camaraderie, shared engagement, and shared anecdotes. Also, mealtimes are infinitely more comfortable if you eat with someone who understands the basics of the plan.

There are also many discussions in online discussion forums. Mums nets are an excellent source of support and information. It is remarkable how reassuring it is to know that you are not alone.

Quick Meal Preparation

Prepare your quick meal in advance, so you do not have to search for food and come across a sausage that irresistibly hides in the fridge. Keep it simple and effortlessly strive for the taste of the day. Buy and cook on non-fast days to avoid snickering at inappropriate temptations. Clean the house of junk food before embarking. It will only sing and coo in the closets, making your fasting day more difficult than it should be.

Check the Partial Size of the Calorie Label

If the cereal box says "30 g," weigh it. Continue. Be surprised. Then be honest. Your calorie count is necessarily fixed and limited on an empty stomach, so it is important not to worry about how much is flowing. Here, you'll find our recommended fast food calorie counters. More importantly, do not count calories on late days.

You have better things. Wait before you eat. Resist at least 10 minutes, and preferably 15 minutes, to see if your hunger subsides (which is usually the case). If you need a snack, choose one that does not raise your insulin levels. Try carrots, a handful of popcorn, apple slices, or strawberries. But do not pinch like chicken all day. Calories are stacked up quickly, and your fasting is fast. Eat consciously on a fasting day and fully absorb the fact that you are eating (especially if you have ever been in a massive traffic jam). Also, be careful with your vacation. Do not eat until you are satisfied (of course, this happens after a few weeks of practice). Find out what the concept of "satisfaction" means to you. We are all different, and it changes over time.

Stay Busy

"We humans are always looking for activities between meals," Leonard Cohen said. Yes, see where it takes us. So, fill your day, not your face. "No one is hungry during the first few seconds of skydiving," said Brad Pilon, the advocate of fasting. Distraction is the best defense against the dark art of the food industry, with doughnuts and nachos on every corner. If you need this doughnut, keep in mind that it will remain tomorrow.

Try 2 to 2

Fast from 2:00 p.m. to 2:00 p.m., not from bedtime to bedtime. After lunch on the first day, eat modestly until lunch on the next day.

This way, you will lose weight during sleep and will not feel uncomfortable for a day without food. This is a smart trick, but it requires a bit more focus than the all-day option. Alternatively, you can go from dinner to dinner quickly. In short, no day is fast and fun. The point is that this plan is "adapted to adjustment." Just like your waist.

Get Started

Determine the Start Date

We strongly recommend starting on Monday. It makes more sense. After you have selected a day, you can thoroughly prepare for the start time with a few steps.

Select the Distribution of Fast/Meal to Determine When to Eat and Fast

16/8 is recommended for beginners. You don't have to get used to it a lot, and it is not too difficult the first time. Select a window and decide when to stop eating the night before fasting. It will serve as a separate house. We recommend that you stick to it for the first week. After practicing IF for a few weeks, it is only natural to change windows and schedules. However, it is best to keep the same time during the first week. So, if you stop eating at 9 p.m. on Sunday, you won't eat at 1 p.m. on Monday. From 1 p.m. to 9 p.m., it will be an eating window.

Spend a Flirt Day

Spend one day on the day before the first fast. Eat a lot and eat whatever you like. It has two purposes. First, the more foods there are in the system, the easier it is to make fast first. Secondly, if you eat the things you want the night before, that means you won't thirst for these foods for a week.

Teach People

I highly recommend talking to your loved ones about the new habits you are adopting. Explain why you do it and why you are committed—politely informed them that you do not eat at certain times and that you will like their support, please. Warn people to make up for your chances of getting food during a fast. One of the most difficult challenges you face is that of a friend, family, or colleague who provides you with food—tell about your IF and avoid it.

Buy Branched-Chain Amino Acids (Optional)

Branched-chain amino acids (BCAA) are beneficial on an empty stomach. These are pure forms of protein and incredibly powerful for more prolonged fasting. Consuming 10 g of BCAAs can help reduce hunger without fasting. Do not exceed 10 g per serving, but two servings are enough during fasting. If you want to exercise, I recommend BCAA. If you are going to exercise, we recommend that you exercise 60 minutes before and during exercise at one of the following times:

Training and Intermittent Fasting

You do not have to exercise to take advantage of intermittent fasting. However, when you select training, you'll see unprecedented levels of results. As explained earlier in this book, IF increases growth hormone and testosterone production and attacks adipocytes and stores. With the addition of an exercise routine (we recommend strength training), the results you see are incredible. Strength training combined with increased hormones can help you build muscle faster than expected. Lifting weights also increases the production of testosterone and growth hormone, so your body receives twice the dose of hormone production. Weight training is also very metabolic, so shred fat from your body and remember, as I said, you have more muscles, which means less fat.

I would also like to mention that strength training and exercise are probably the most effective way to protect your body from whatever the world throws at you. It has been proven to reduce stress, help with depression, increase energy levels, improve mental function, increase your happiness, improve your life, and help you live longer. Therefore, it is highly recommended to start training. If you do not have a good gym, strength exercises like pushups, squats, and lunges can help you on your journey. Finally, I would like to add one thing, if it can be speeded up, run it. I understand that planning does not mean everyone can do it, but one way to improve is to exercise and fast with a meal after exercise. Do not eat more than 2 hours after weight training, as your muscles will be disrupted, and this will negatively affect your goals.

Chapter 8:   Foods to Eat and to Avoid

Food always plays a very important role in our overall health. The health debacle that we are facing these days has two important parts:

- Our Eating Habits
- The Things We Eat

Our Eating Habits

This is a very important part because poor eating habits and reckless eating can damage our whole food processing and energy management system. Intermittent fasting is the answer to poor eating habits as it can help you in improving your food intake.

This is helpful to a great extent. Intermittent fasting relies on managing your eating habits to such a great extent that if you can manage your eating habits properly, you can eat anything you like in moderation.

This might seem to be a great exaggeration for the people who have been following punishing diets all their lives. Cycles of restrictions, endless temptations, and events of binge eating are the major phases in their lives.

Intermittent fasting doesn't pose such restrictions. If you are feeling compelled to eat the cake your friend is offering you, you may go ahead and have a bite of it in your eating window without developing any guilt. This is not to say that cake is not unhealthy. It is made up of refined carbs, refined sugar, and unhealthy fats. However, as long as you are eating it in moderation, you will be able to avoid major issues in your weight loss journey.

A big reason women on punishing diets are not able to lose weight is their endless temptation for the forbidden things. It is very human to desire the things that you can't have, especially food. Diets put too many restrictions, and hence the dieters always feel tempted, and that poses emotional, physical, and psychological challenges. They can't eat anything they like without feeling the guilt inside them. Intermittent fasting frees you from any such guilt. It allows you to eat the things you like in moderation so that there is no long-term temptation that may lead to binge eating or psychological barriers in the end.

The Things We Eat

The things we eat do play a role in our health. You can offset the harmful effects of some food products by not consuming them in large quantities but that doesn't make them good or healthy.

- There are limited things that you should eat in good quantities.

- There are a few things that you may only eat in moderation.
- There are a few things that you must avoid.

Macronutrients

Fat, proteins, and carbohydrates are the three macronutrients and you must have them in balanced quantities. Trapped in our fast-paced lives, we seldom pay attention to the macronutrients in food and their importance in our health. If you do not consume the three macronutrients in healthy proportions, you may find it very difficult to control your hunger, cravings, and energy levels. Imbalanced intake of these macronutrients can also lead to faster satiety and faster hunger pangs. You may also feel energy drained.

If you want to follow a healthy intermittent fasting routine, you must have a balanced meal in the following proportions.

Fat: 50-70%

The fat must constitute the highest part of your diet if you want to lose weight faster and have a better fasting routine. This may sound counterproductive as you are trying to lose fat, but there is no relation between eating healthy fat and gaining fat. On the condition that you are consuming healthy fats within your calorie limits, you will be losing weight just fine. Not only this, but healthy fats are also beneficial in lowering the risk of heart disorders and chronic inflammations.

- Nuts and Seeds: Almonds, walnuts, flax seeds, chia seeds, are great sources of healthy fats
- Fatty fish: Wild-caught fatty fish provides a lot of healthy fat. They are also a rich source of Omega3 fatty acids.
- Eggs: Egg is among the finest sources of fats. The egg yolk provides very healthy fat and can be consumed safely.
- Avocado: It is also a very good source of healthy fat.
- Olive oil: It is a good option to be used for cooking. However, even using too much olive oil can be harmful. You must use it in moderation.

Fat in your diet should be the highest if you want your body to get into ketosis. If you keep consuming too many carbs, even though your calorie intake may remain low you'd always face difficulty in burning fat.

Another difficulty in consuming too many carbs is that they burn faster and you may start having cravings too fast and remaining in the fasting state may become difficult. The fat is a slow-burning fuel and hence it takes much longer to get processed and hence you wouldn't feel hunger pangs fast.

Protein: 15-25%

Protein in the diet is very significant as our body can't produce protein. You will have to consume protein to compensate for all the loss of tissues, muscles, and the structural repair work in the body. Therefore, it is a macronutrient that isn't optional. However, although protein is so important, you can't have a lot of it.

If you are not doing serious physical work that involves a lot of muscle or tissue damage, your protein requirements would be moderate. Any excess protein consumed would be converted to carbs and hence, there would be an imbalance in your diet.

You can get healthy proteins from:

- Lean meats
- Legumes
- Pulses
- Egg whites
- White meat poultry
- Lean cuts of meat
- Soy
- Seafood

Striking a healthy balance with protein is very important. It can be crucial to your fasting routine as well. Protein takes the longest to get processed in the gut, and hence it keeps your digestive system engaged. If you are consuming protein in a balanced manner, you are less likely to feel hungry very often.

Carbohydrate 5-10%

Carbs are a major part of the modern diet. Our diet is filled with refined flours, refined sugar, processed food items, etc. They have a lot of carbs. Not only this, but most of our staple food items are also carb-rich, and hence we feel trapped when we are asked to lower our carb intake.

However, this is a mental limitation we have created. There are a lot of carbs that are healthy and can be consumed without any limitation.

Within carbs, there is a distinction between good carbs and bad carbs, and you must keep that distinction in mind.

Bad Carbs

- All Refined Flours: You must not consume food items made up of refined flours. You must make it a practice to read the food labels carefully.

- Refined Sugar: Things made up of refined sugar must be eliminated from the diet. They will lead to food cravings and cause serious health issues.
- Empty Calories: This is the third category you must stay away from. All the processed items that are made up of maple syrup, fructose, or sugar, must be avoided at all costs. You must also avoid carbonated beverages, sweetened beverages, fruit juices, and even fresh fruit juices. Most people have a misconception in their minds that fresh fruit juices are nutritious, but they are wrong. They only have calories and some vitamins, but they are devoid of all the minerals that your body needed. You must also avoid alcohol or other such things that have lots of concentrated carbs.

These things lead to a glucose spike in your bloodstream, invoking an immediate and heavy insulin response, but they do not offer anything to your gut. Your gut starts releasing gastric juices in anticipation but gets nothing in return. As a result, you may develop acid reflux, ulcer, and other such issues. The glucose spike in your bloodstream is also temporary as your body lowers the glucose level rapidly, and you soon start feeling the urge to have something to eat.

This is a reason you feel very good when you eat sugar-rich foods, but start feeling energy devoid very soon.

Good Carbs

Whole Grains: Whole grains are undoubtedly great for your gut as well as your body, and you must have them in smaller quantities. Whole grains have a lot of trace minerals that are important for your body, and you can't get them from other sources. Apart from that, they are a rich source of indigestible fiber that is very helpful in scrubbing your intestines clean.

- Non-starchy Leafy Greens: You can have non-starchy leafy greens as much as you want without thinking about your calorie intake. They are full of vitamins and antioxidants. Leafy greens are filling, and hence they will keep your stomach occupied without providing too many calories, and you wouldn't even feel hungry very often. Apart from that, leafy greens are full of soluble fiber that gets converted into a gel-like substance in your gut and cleanses your digestive system softly. It is very helpful and hence, must be consumed in good quantities.
- Salads and Fruits: You can have salads and fruits in healthy quantities as they are also a rich source of fiber. You must try to have as much fiber as possible because it keeps your digestive system engaged, clean, and healthy.

Chapter 9:   Mistakes to Avoid in Intermittent Fasting

Now that you know all about the process of intermittent fasting and how it should be done, you should also know the common mistakes that people make while fasting. These mistakes can actually prevent you from realizing the benefits and make the entire fast nothing, but a complete waste. So, once you know what they are, make sure that you do not make the same mistakes yourself. If you do not want to make mistakes, the first and foremost thing that you need to do is be aware of everything that you are doing and also know why you are doing them. This will ensure that even if you are sometimes off the path, you can easily push yourself back on track. Also, stop beating yourself up for a cheat day or any mistake that you made. Just move on by accepting that it happened, and it cannot be undone. If you waste your energy in self-loathing, you will not be able to make plans so that the same mistake does not happen twice.

Fasting Too Long Even at the Beginning

You must have heard me saying this plenty of times already; you need to take it slow. Do not rush the process. If you haven't tried intermittent fasting ever in your life, then you should start with a 48-hour fast or even a 24-hour fast for that matter. Yes, you will have to eventually lengthen the fasting window, but that does not mean you have to do it now and at once. What you have to do is increase the fasting period but do it in small increments. In case you do not follow what I said, it will be you who will be facing certain consequences and they are bound to happen.

One of the first consequences that people have to face when they fast for longer periods too quickly is that they become grumpy. They behave badly with coworkers and loved ones. And the worst part is that you might shove it away, saying that it's just your way of coping with fasting, but it is not. Also, due to your cranky mood, some people might even give you negative feedback, and in most cases, that is when people give up the fast and throw every effort down the gutter all at once. Tossing the whole idea out of the window because of such a situation is not worth it and it wouldn't have come to it only if you had increased your fasting period gradually.

The second consequence is that when people do longer fast, in the beginning, they cannot continue it after the first couple of days mainly because it becomes too unbearable for them, and they feel tremendously hungry all the time. The process of intermittent fasting should not make you feel jarred or stressed. Instead, it should be gradual and gentle. If you truly want to continue intermittent fasting for a long stretch of time, you have to learn to make it well incorporated into your routine and for that, you need to take it slow. When you start the longer fasts right from the beginning, you are simply walking on the path of disappointment and most people give up too quickly in such cases.

Not Eating the Right Foods

This is probably the biggest mistake that I see people have been making. If you have been trying to incorporate the process of intermittent fasting into your day-to-day life, then you also have to ensure that you are eating the right foods; otherwise, it won't work the way you want it to. For starters, as you might know, fasting means that you have to learn how to get your appetite under control. And this means that you cannot simply grab that packet of chips or that bar of crunchy granola whenever you feel like it. There is a time for everything, and time is highly essential. But equally essential is what you are eating in your eating window.

If you make the wrong choices, then you are definitely going to have a hard time controlling your appetite. When you are relying on foods that are rich in carbohydrates, you will be deliberately making the entire process difficult for yourself; your appetite along with your levels of blood glucose are in a state of continuous fluctuation. When you are on a diet that is low in carbs, you will have more fats and proteins. This will increase your levels of satiety. In simpler words, you will remain full for a longer period of time. Moreover, this will give your body flexibility in metabolism so that you can tap into your fat reserves whenever your body is fasting and does not have enough glucose as fuel.

Also, some people use intermittent fasting as an excuse to eat whatever they want when they are in the eating window. That is not right and won't bring you any good results. You have to remember that this is not a magic pill, and nothing will happen on its own if you do not put in enough effort. It is true that intermittent fasting allows you to take your health into your own hands and maintain proper metabolism but for that, your diet needs to be healthy too. You have to cut down on sugar and processed foods. You need to incorporate more and more whole foods that are rich in nutrients and low in carbs.

Consuming Too Many Calories

It is important to eat the right foods so that you can get the nutrients that you need. But you should not overdo it in the eating phase. When people fast, they have this idea that they have to replenish themselves by eating an equally heavy meal in the eating window. Never try to compensate for the time you were not eating. Sometimes people end up overeating to such an extent that they not only regret their actions, but also feel bloated.

Also, in case you have overeaten, don't be too harsh on yourself because it will only make matters worse. Accept that fact, because you simply cannot undo it in any way. What you have to do from now on is that you have to prepare and plan your meals and keep healthy options in every meal. This will ensure that when the eating window starts, you don't have to think about what you want to eat. A very important part of the process of intermittent fasting is to figure out a balance in your routine where you can prepare healthy foods and not depend on processed foods.

Not Staying Consistent

This is probably true for everything on earth that if you are not consistent with it, it will not bring you results. The same goes for intermittent fasting. But what is worse is that if you are not consistent, then you will be stuck in a cycle where you make poor eating choices and you will be so disappointed with everything that you will not feel like doing anything about it. That is exactly something you need to avoid and for this, you have to be consistent. The best way to ensure this is to follow a fasting regime that you can maintain for the long term. You need to understand that if you truly want to reap the benefits of intermittent fasting, then it also means that you have to do it for a long period of time without giving up on it.

In case you already feel like that, you will not be able to stay consistent throughout the procedure, then you need to sit down and figure out why. You need to find the reason behind it and then deal with it. Is it because you do not like the method that you have selected? If it is so, then try some other method. Or is it because you're fasting and feeding window is wrong and you are having a hard time adjusting to it? In that case, you need to adjust the timings in a different manner. Whatever it is, just don't give up before figuring out the why.

Doing Too Many Things at the Same Time

This is also one of the reasons why people give up on intermittent fasting, especially beginners. There is a saying that you should not bite off more than you can chew, and this is exactly what I am talking about here. If you are trying out intermittent fasting for the first time and you are also trying to maintain a daily gym schedule (which you don't usually do) and on top that, you are also trying to cook your own meals (when you are habituated to take-outs), then it is very easy to feel stressed.

So, maybe you can start by training only three times a week and then you can take the help of your family members in cooking your meals. If you do not have anyone living with you, then you can skip the gym for now and maybe go for a run in the neighborhood in the initial days. Once you are okay with this routine, then you can incorporate the gym.

Now that you know the common mistakes, I hope this will help you to avoid them.

Chapter 10: Exercise and Intermittent Fasting to Lose Weight

Many people will ask if it is safe to combine fasting with exercise. I am here to say it is. However, some factors need to be considered before combining the two. First, the type of fasting regimen should be considered alongside the physical, mental, and psychological health of the individual. Women with existing medical conditions should not combine fasting with exercises before being advised by a medical expert. So, while it is safe to practice intermittent fasting and include exercise if you are an already active person, doing so is not suitable for everyone.

First of all, your metabolism can be negatively impacted if you exercise and fast for long periods. For example, if you exercise daily while fasting for more than a month, your metabolic rate can begin to slow down. So, while it may sound like a quick way to reap the benefits of your limited calorie intake, moderation is crucial.

Combining the two can trigger a higher rate of breaking down glycogen and body fat. This means that you burn fat at an accelerated rate. Also, when you combine these two, your growth hormones are boosted. This results in improved bone density. Your muscles are also positively impacted when you exercise. Your muscles will become more resilient to stress and age slower. This is also a quick way to trigger autophagy keeping brain cells and tissues strong, making you feel and look younger.

Exercise is Even Better After 50

Cardiovascular exercise is great for the heart and lungs. It improves oxygen delivery to specific parts of your body, reduces stress, improves sleep, burns fat, and improves sex drive. Some of the more common cardio exercises are running, brisk walking, and swimming. In the gym, machines such as the elliptical, treadmill, and Stairmaster are used to help with cardio. Some people are satisfied and feel like they've done enough after 20 minutes on the treadmill, but if you want to continue to be strong and independent as you grow older, you need to consider adding strength training to your workout. After 50, strength training for a woman is no longer about six-pack abs, building biceps, or vanity muscles. Instead, it has switched to maintaining a body that is healthy, strong, and is less prone to injury and illness.

Women over 50 who engage in strength training for 20 to 30 minutes a day can reap the following benefits:

- Reduced body fat: Accumulating excess body fat is not healthy for any woman at any age. To prevent many of the diseases associated with aging, it is important to maintain healthy body weight by burning excess fat.
- Build bone density: With stronger bones, accidental falls are less likely to result in broken limbs or a visit to the emergency room.

- Build muscle mass: Although you are not likely to be the next champion bodybuilder, strength training will make you an overall stronger woman who will carry herself with ease, push your lawnmower, lift your groceries, and perform all other tasks that require you to exert some strength.
- Significant less risk of chronic diseases: In addition to keeping chronic diseases away, strength training can also reduce symptoms of some diseases you may have, such as back pain, obesity, arthritis, osteoporosis, and diabetes. Of course, the type of exercises you do if you have any chronic disease should be recommended by your doctor.
- Boosts mental health: A loss of self-confidence and depression are some psychological issues that come along with aging. Women who keep themselves fit with exercises tend to be generally more self-assured and are less likely to develop depression.

Strength Training Exercises for Women Over 50

These ten-strength training exercises you can do right in the comfort of your home. All you need is a mat, a chair, and some hand weights of about 3-8 pounds. As you get stronger, you can increase the weight. Take a minute to rest before switching between each routine. Ensure that you move slowly through the exercises, breathe properly, and focus on maintaining the right form. If you start to feel lightheaded or dizzy during your routines, especially if you are performing the exercise during your fasting window, stop immediately.

Squat to Chair

This exercise is great for improving your bone health. A lot of age-related bone fractures and falls in women involve the pelvis, so this exercise will target and strengthen your pelvic bone and the surrounding muscles.
To perform this:
1. Stand fully upright in front of a chair as if you are ready to sit and spread your feet shoulder-width apart.
2. Extend your arms in front of you and keep them that way all through the movement.
3. Bend your knees and slowly lower your hips as if you want to sit on the chair, but don't sit. When your butt touches the chair slightly, press into your heels to get back your initial standing position. Repeat that about 10 to 15 times.

Forearm Plank

This exercise targets your core and shoulders.
Here's how to do it:

1. Get into a push-up position, but with your arms bent at the elbows such that your forearm is supporting your weight.
2. Keep your body off the mat or floor and keep your back straight at all times. Don't raise or drop your hips. This will engage your core. Hold the position for 30 seconds and then drop to your knees. Repeat ten times.

Modified Push-Ups

This routine targets your arms, shoulders, and core.

How's how to do it:
1. Kneel on your mat. Place your hands on the mat below your shoulders and let your knees be behind your hips so that your back is stretched at an angle.
2. Tuck your toes under and tighten your abdominal muscles. Gradually bend your elbows as you lower your chest toward the floor.
3. Push back on your arms to press your chest back to your earlier position. Repeat as many times as is comfortable.

Bird Dog

When done correctly, this exercise can strengthen the muscles of your posterior chain as it targets your back and core. It may seem easy at first, but can be a bit tricky.

To do this correctly:
1. Go on all fours on your mat.
2. Tighten your abdominal muscles and shift your weight to your right knee and left hand. Slowly extend your right hand in front of you and your left leg behind you. Ensure that both your hands and legs are extended as far as possible and stay in that position for about 5 seconds. Return to your starting position. This is one repetition. Switch to your left knee and right hand and repeat the movement. Alternate between both sides for 20 repetitions.

Shoulder Overhead Press

This targets your biceps, shoulders, and back.

To perform this move:
1. With dumbbells in both hands, stand and spread your feet shoulder-width apart.
2. Bring the dumbbells up to the sides of your head and tighten your abdominal muscles.
3. Slowly press the dumbbells up until your arms are straight above your head. Slowly return to the first position. Repeat 10 times. You can also do this exercise while sitting.

Chest Fly

This targets your chest, back, core, and glutes.

To do this:

1. Lie with your back flat on your mat, your knees at an angle close to 90 degrees, and your feet firmly planted on the floor or mat.
2. Hold dumbbells in both hands over your chest. Keep your palms facing each other and gently open your hands away from your chest. Let your upper arms touch the floor without releasing the tension in them.
3. Contract your chest muscles and slowly return the dumbbells to the initial position. Repeat about ten times.

Standing Calf Raise

This exercise improves the mobility of your lower legs and feet and also improves your stability. Here's how to perform it.

1. Hold a dumbbell in your left hand and place your right hand on something sturdy to give you balance.
2. When you are sure of your balance, lift your left foot off the floor with the dumbbell hanging at your side. Stand erect and move your weight such that you are almost standing on your toes.
3. Slowly return to the starting position. Do this 15 times before switching to the other leg and doing the same thing all over again.

Single-Leg Hamstring Bridge

This move targets your glutes, quads, and hamstrings.

To do this:

1. Lie flat on your back. Place your feet flat on the floor or mat and spread your bent knees apart.
2. Place your arms flat by your side and lift one leg straight.
3. Contract your glutes as you lift your hips into a bridge position with your arms still in position. Hold for about 2 to 3 seconds and drop your hips to the mat. Repeat about ten times before switching your leg. Do the same again.

Bent-Over Row

This targets your back muscles and spine.

To do this:

1. Hold dumbbells in both hands and stand behind a sturdy object (for example, a chair). Bend forward and rest your head on the chosen object. Relax your neck and slightly bend your knees. With both palms facing each other pull the dumbbells to touch your ribs. Hold the position for about 2 to 5 seconds and slowly return to the starting position. Repeat 10 to 15 times.

Basic Ab

A distended belly is a common occurrence in older women. This exercise can strengthen and tighten the abdominal muscles bringing them inward toward your spine.

To perform this:

1. Lie on your back with your feet firmly planted on the floor and your knees bent. Relax your upper body and rest your hands on your thighs.
2. As you exhale, lift yourself upward off the mat or floor. Stop the upward movement when your hands are resting on your knees. Hold the position for about 2 to 5 seconds and then slowly return to the starting position. Repeat for about 20 to 30 times.

Include Exercises in Your Daily Routine

You do not have to hit the gym or plan a time dedicated to working out. You can make exercise part of your daily routine so that you are always getting the proper amount of body movement, whether or not it is time for exercise.

Here are a few tips on how to include exercises into your daily routine.

- Take the stairs (within reason) instead of using the elevator. You don't want to go up a ten-story building using the stairs! If you have a long way to go up or down, take the stairs a couple of flights and then complete your trip with the elevator.
- When you talk with your family members at home, don't shout from the top floor and bottom floor. Go up or climb down and talk with them.
- Find a sporting activity that you thoroughly enjoy and do it as often as is convenient. When you're doing something you enjoy, you'll hardly think of it as exercise, and you're likely to stay committed.
- If you are at work, instead of sending emails or text messages to coworkers, walk up to them and talk to them face to face.
- If possible, convert your one-on-one meetings to a walking meeting. Hold the meeting while taking a stroll outside.
- Stop a block or two from your destination and walk the rest of the way. Make walking your preferred mode of transportation.
- Take your dog for walks daily. If you don't have a dog, adopt one. It might seem that you are merely walking your dog, but you are exercising your muscles.

- Take brisk walks as often as possible. Remember to put on comfortable shoes when walking briskly. You can bring your walking shoes with you to make it easy for you to change into them.

Staying Safe While Combining Intermittent Fasting and Exercise

Exercising in your fasting window can help you quickly achieve some of the advanced benefits of intermittent fasting. Nevertheless, it is crucial to follow a few general guidelines to keep you safe during the practice.

There are no iron-cast rules about when to exercise even on fasting days. Observe what works well for you—whether exercising before eating (during the fasting window) or eating before working out (during the eating window). Many women find that exercising on an empty stomach suits their bodies, and leaves them feeling energized for the rest of the day. If this is your case, set aside time in the morning before your first meal of the day. Some other women find that although they prefer working out on an empty stomach, they feel depleted right after the exercise. In that case, shift your exercise to about 20 to 30 minutes before your first meal of the day. Your body would have rested a bit after your exercise before you breakfast.

If you prefer working out after you breakfast, that is perfectly fine. Eating shortly before your exercise doesn't render your exercises ineffective. Remember that all of our bodies work in different ways.

Keep in mind that the goal of working out is to maintain proper body health long into your golden years. You don't need to impress anyone with great abs or biceps, instead impress yourself with how much power you have. Stay committed to your routines, but don't overdo it. If you start feeling weak, that is your cue to take a break.

If you are fasting for longer periods (24 hours or more), you will need to conserve your energy. Consider doing exercises that will not exert too much stress. Take a walk, do some yoga or any other type of low-intensity exercise.

We could all use someone on our shoulder reminding us to drink more water. And going without food reduces your body's water content even more. Add higher levels of exertion and you'll be depleting your water reserves very quickly. So here is your reminder to always drink adequate amounts of water before, during, and after your workout sessions.

Chapter 11: Tips to Overcome Down Moment During Fasting

Alright, so you want to start doing this fasting thing, but you have some concerns. "Won't I be starving and irritable?" "I don't want to go to jail for work-place violence..."

Fortunately for you, after a week or so, the hunger pangs you usually have in the morning will shift to lunchtime (or later). But to make it easier, here are some strategies you can use to make you an IF master.

Black Coffee

If you're like me, you drink coffee every morning so that this one will be easy for you. If you can drink it black, this will keep your body in a fasted state. If you put milk or cream in it, your body will start to use that for energy instead of your body fat. Which would you rather occur? The other benefit of coffee is that it blunts hunger. Try it, if you feel hungry, drink a cup or two of black coffee and see how you feel. I find it elevates my focus, so I become a machine at work. No, not a robot, but a highly effective, clear-minded beast! There are some hidden benefits related to caffeine increasing the amount of fat you burn. At the same time, you've fasted, but you can find those with a simple google search. We aren't here to waste your time with citations. As usual, I like to stick with the more practical and obvious benefits, and those are hunger blunting and increasing productivity. Try it; you'll love it.

Seltzer Water

This one is similar to coffee—if you start to feel a little hungry, a little empty in the belly, try drinking a can of sparkling water. The zero-calorie kind that is flavored is my favorite. I drink this cran-raspberry version from La Croix. The carbonation seems to take up space in your belly and kills hunger. I also just like to have a nice fizzy drink from time to time. Freshwater is excellent, but sometimes while I'm working, it's refreshing to sip a flavored beverage.

A Piece of Fruit

Okay, so let's say you have made it to lunchtime fasted, but you'd like to push it a little further. Sometimes, I want to try my first meal a bit further into the afternoon, like 3-5 pm, but at this point, you're going to start feeling hungry, and it's time to eat. For me, though, I'm sometimes so focused on work that I'd instead not cook. Now is the time to grab a piece of fruit from the fridge. Maybe an apple or a peach.

As I mentioned in regards to putting milk in your coffee, this will shift your body out of fasting mode, but that's okay, the point of eating now is, again, to blunt your hunger so that you have even more calories. Maybe it's a holiday, and you're planning to let loose at the dinner table.

Use these strategies to have a large-enough calorie buffer that you can eat all you want and still lose weight! Remember though, that you aren't trying to starve yourself, and if at any point you start to feel irritable or begin to notice a decline in your work, eat. Listen to your body. For me, if I sometimes want to push my first meal until after work, I might start feeling a bit anxious towards the end of the day, so the fruit brings me back on point.

Meal Sizing

This last strategy is how you choose to split your meals' size and is more of a personal preference. It would help if you determined what works best for you.

• One Large Meal and One Smaller Meal

The one-large-and-one-small-meal strategy is what I've been using because it allows me to have a massive meal for my first meal, which honestly keeps me satisfied to the point where I usually don't feel much hunger for the rest of the day. I like it because it has simplified my life so much. I only have to prepare one meal per day, and then my second meal is practically a snack—a couple of small quesadillas or a few eggs and a piece of toast. And if you wanted to, you could swap your meals so the first one is small and then your dinnertime meal is the big one. Perfect for saving up your calories for a dinner date.

• Two Medium-Sized Meals

I once followed this strategy for a very long time, and its most significant benefit is maintenance. If you like the weight you are at and want to maintain it, have two medium-sized meals. What's a medium-sized meal? It's the usual amount of food you would eat for lunch or dinner, a standard plate of food. You can even follow this plan to lose weight too, since you'll be cutting out breakfast and eating less. I tended not to lose weight because, as I mentioned earlier, I like food like a little too much. So, my medium was a powerful medium.

- ## Three Smaller Meals

Everyone is different, and some people are grazers. You like to munch on things here and there. A small salad here, maybe a granola bar, some fancy vegan cookies. Now, I'm not advocating cookies, but I know people that just don't eat big meals. It's too much for them. If they ate as I did, they would be on the floor in pain. The Three-Small-Meals plan is perfect for them. You've shifted your calories to the afternoon. By eating as usual, you'll have once again achieved that calorie deficit (eating less) you need to lose weight. The problem with this style is that you might overeat. At some point, you need to know exactly how much food you put in your body on a typical day. Overeaters tend to eat more carb-centric or sugary things, which your body uses up fast, leaving you hungry again quickly. That's why I suggest trying to eat a larger meal with the right amount of fat to keep you nice and full. If it works for you, though, then do it. Keep an eye on your weight and, if you see progress, you're good to go!

Chapter 12: Healthy Recipes - Breakfast

1. Avocado Egg Bowls

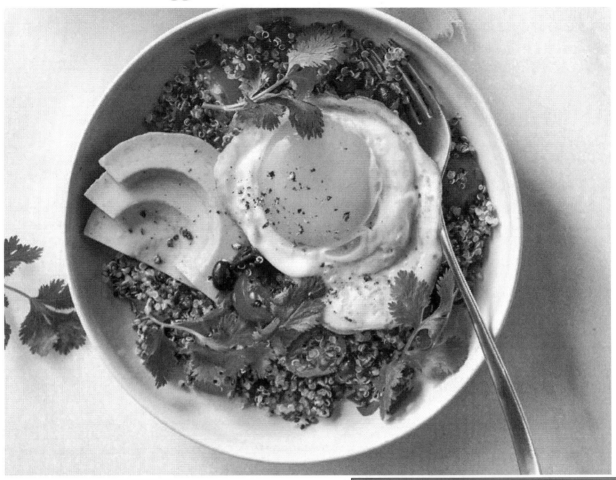

Preparation Time: 5 Minutes
Cooking Time: 10 Minutes
Servings: 3

- Chopped walnuts
- Balsamic Pearls
- Fresh thyme

Ingredients:

- 1 tsp. of coconut oil
- 2 organics eggs, free-range
- Salt and pepper
- 1 large and ripe avocado

For Garnishing:

Directions:

1. Slice your avocado in two, then take out the pit and remove enough of the inside so that there is enough space inside to accommodate an entire egg.
2. Cut off a little bit of the bottom of the avocado so that the avocado will sit upright as you place it on a stable surface.

3. Open your eggs and put each of the yolks in a separate bowl or container. Place the egg whites in the same small bowl. Sprinkle some pepper and salt to the whites, according to your taste, then mix them well.
4. Melt the coconut oil in a pan that has a lid that fits and put it on med-high.
5. Put in the avocado boats, with the meaty side down on the pan, the skin side up and sauté them for approx. 35 seconds or when they become darker in color.
6. Turn them over, then add to the spaces inside, almost filling the inside with the whites of the eggs.
7. Then, reduce the temperature and place the lid. Let them sit covered for approx. 16 to 20 minutes until the whites are just about fully cooked.
8. Gently add one yolk onto each of the avocados and keep cooking them for 4 to 5 minutes, just until they get to the point of cook you want them at.
9. Move the avocados to a dish and add toppings to each of them using the walnuts, the balsamic pearls, or/and thyme.

Nutrition:

- Calories: 215 kcal
- Total Fat: 18g
- Carbohydrates: 8g
- Protein: 9g

2. Buttery Date Pancakes

Preparation Time: 10 Minutes
Cooking Time: 10 Minutes
Servings: 3

Ingredients:

- 1/4 cup of almond flour
- 3 eggs, beaten
- 1 tsp. of olive oil
- 6 dates, pitted
- 1 tbsp. of almond butter
- 1 tsp. of vanilla extract
- 1/2 tsp. of ground cinnamon

Directions:

1. Stir the eggs in a bowl to make them fluffy.
2. Wash the dates and cut them in half.
3. Discard the seeds and mash them finely.
4. Melt the almond butter and add to the eggs.
5. Add the almond flour, olive oil, and cinnamon.
6. Mix well and add the vanilla extract.
7. Mix into a smooth batter.
8. Add the date paste and mix well.
9. In a pan, heat the butter over medium heat.
10. Add the batter using a spoon and fry them golden brown from both sides.
11. Repeat with all the batter.
12. Serve with melted butter on top.

Nutrition:

- Calories: 281 kcal
- Total Fat: 20g
- Carbohydrates: 4.5g,
- Protein: 10.5g

3. Low Carb Pancake Crepes

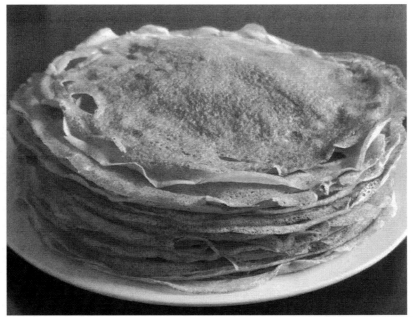

Preparation Time: 10 Minutes
Cooking Time: 10 Minutes
Servings: 2

Ingredients:

- 3 ounces cream cheese
- 1 tsp. of ground cinnamon
- 1 tbsp. of honey
- 1 tsp. of ground cardamom
- 1 tsp. of butter
- 2 eggs, beaten

Directions:

1. In a bowl, whisk the eggs finely.
2. Beat the cream cheese in a different bowl until it becomes soft.
3. Add the egg mixture to the softened cream cheese and mix well until there are no lumps left.
4. Add cinnamon, cardamom, and honey to it. Mix well. The batter would be runnier than pancake batter.
5. In a pan, add the butter and heat over medium heat.
6. Add the batter using a scooper; that way, all the crepes would be the same size.
7. Fry them golden brown on both sides.
8. Repeat the process with the rest of the batter.
9. Drizzle some honey on top and enjoy.

Nutrition:

- Calories: 241 kcal
- Total Fat: 21.8 g
- Carbohydrates: 2.4g
- Protein: 9.6 g

4. Bacon Egg & Sausage Cups

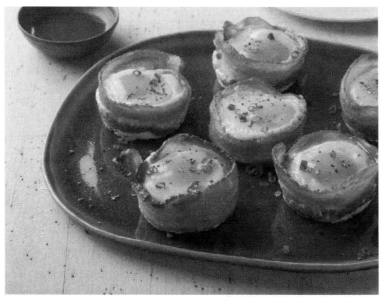

Preparation Time: 10 Minutes
Cooking Time: 20 Minutes
Servings: 8

Ingredients:

- 3 oz. of breakfast sausages
- 2 slices of bacon, chopped
- 4 large eggs
- 2 large green onions, chopped
- 1 oz. of cheddar cheese, shredded
- 1 tbsp. of coconut oil

Directions:

1. Preheat oven to 350°F.
2. Grease your muffin pan and set it aside.
3. In a mixing bowl, beat the eggs together with the cheese. Set it aside.
4. Brown the bacon in a non-stick skillet over medium heat. Add the crumbled sausage and cook until it's no longer pink.
5. Add the onion and cook until wilted. Remove the skillet from the heat and let it cool for a minute or two.
6. Add the meat mixture to the egg mixture and beat well using a spoon.
7. Scoop mixture into the greased muffin pan and bake for 15-20 minutes or until the tops begin to brown. Remove from pan and serve.

Nutrition:

- Calories: 100 kcal
- Fat: 8g
- Fiber: 2g
- Carbs: 20g
- Protein: 5g

5. Chia Seed Banana Blueberry Delight

Preparation Time: 30 Minutes
Cooking Time: 0 Minutes
Servings: 2

Ingredients:

- 1 cup yogurt
- ½ cup blueberries
- 1/2 tsp. Salt
- 1/2 tsp. Cinnamon
- 1 banana
- 1 tsp. Vanilla Extract
- 1/4 cup Chia Seeds

Directions:

1. Discard the skin of the banana.
2. Cut into semi-thick circles.
3. You can mash them or keep them as a whole if you like to bite into your fruits.
4. Clean the blueberries properly and rinse well.
5. Soak the chia seeds in water for 30 minutes or longer.
6. Drain the chia seeds and transfer them into a bowl.
7. Add the yogurt and mix well.
8. Add the salt, cinnamon, and vanilla, and mix again.
9. Now fold in the bananas and blueberries gently.
10. If you want to add dried fruit or nuts, add it and then serve immediately.
11. This is best served cold.

Nutrition:

- Calories: 260 kcal
- Total Fat: 26.6g
- Carbohydrates: 17.4g
- Protein: 4.1g

6. Morning Meatloaf

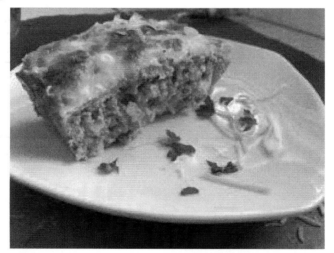

Preparation Time: 10 Minutes
Cooking Time: 20 Minutes

Servings: 6

Ingredients:

- 1 ½ pound of breakfast sausage
- 6 large organic eggs
- 2 tbsp. of unsweetened non-dairy milk
- 1 small onion, finely chopped
- 2 medium garlic cloves, peeled and minced
- 4-ounces of cream cheese softened and cubed
- 1 cup of shredded cheddar cheese
- 2 tbsp. of scallions, chopped
- 1 cup of water

Directions:

1. Add all the ingredients apart from water in a large bowl. Stir until well combined.
2. Form the sausage mixture into a meatloaf and wrap it with a sheet of aluminum foil.

Ensure that the meatloaf fits inside your Instant Pot. If not, remove parts of the mixture and reserve for future use.
3. Once you wrap the meatloaf into a packet, add 1 cup of water and a trivet to your Instant Pot. Put the meatloaf on the trivet's top.
4. Cover and cook for 25 minutes on high pressure. When done, quickly release the pressure. Carefully remove the lid.
5. Unwrap the meatloaf and check if the meatloaf is done. Serve and enjoy!

Nutrition:

- Calories: 592 kcal
- Total Fat: 49.5g
- Carbohydrates: 2.5g
- Protein: 11g

7. Savory Breakfast Muffins

Preparation Time: 10 Minutes
Cooking Time: 35 Minutes
Servings: 6

Ingredients:

- 8 eggs
- 1 cup shredded cheese
- Salt and pepper to taste
- ½ tsp. baking powder
- ¼ cup diced onion
- 2/3 cup coconut flour
- 1 ½ cup spinach
- ¼ cup full fat coconut milk
- 1 tbsp. basil, chopped
- ½ cup cooked chicken, diced finely

Directions:

1. Preheat the oven to 375°F.

2. Use butter or oil to grease your muffin tray or you can use muffin paper liners.
3. In a large mixing bowl, whisk the eggs.
4. Add in the coconut milk and mix again.
5. Gradually shift in the coconut flour with baking powder and salt.
6. Add in the cooked chicken, onion, spinach, basil, and combine well.
7. Add the cheese and mix again.
8. Pour the mixture onto your muffin liners.
9. Bake for about 25 minutes.
10. Serve at room temperature.

Nutrition:

- Calories: 388 kcal
- Total Fat: 25.8g
- Carbohydrates: 8.6g
- Protein: 25.3g

8. Low-Carb Brownies

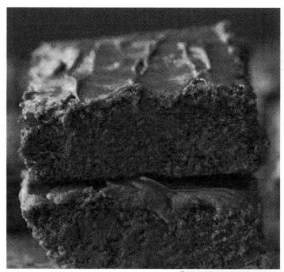

Preparation Time: 10 Minutes
Cooking Time: 20 Minutes
Servings: 16
Ingredients:

- 7 tbsp. of coconut oil, melted
- 6 tbsp. of plant-based sweetener
- 1 large egg
- 2 egg yolks
- 1/2 tsp. of mint extract
- 5 ounces of sugar-free dark chocolate
- ¼ cup of plant-based chocolate protein powder
- 1 tsp. of baking soda
- ¼ tsp. of sea salt
- 2 tbsp. of vanilla almond milk, unsweetened

Directions:

1. Start by preheating the oven to 350°F and then take an 8x8-inch pan and line it with parchment paper, being sure to leave some extra sticking up to use later to help you get them out of the pan after they are cooked.
2. Into a medium-sized vessel, use a hand mixer, and blend 5 tablespoons of the coconut oil (save the rest for later), as well as the egg, Erythritol, egg yolks, and the mint extract all together for 1 minute. After this minute, the mixture will become a lighter yellow hue.
3. Take 4 oz. of the chocolate and put it in a (microwave-safe) bowl, as well as with the other 2 tablespoons of melted coconut oil.
4. Cook this chocolate and oil mixture on half power, at 30-second intervals, being sure to stir at each interval, just until the chocolate becomes melted and smooth
5. While the egg mixture is being beaten, add the melted chocolate mixture into the egg mixture until this becomes thick and homogenous.
6. Add your protein powder of choice, salt, baking soda, and stir until homogenous. Then, vigorously whisk your almond milk in until the batter becomes a bit smoother.

7. Finely chop the rest of your chocolate and stir these bits of chocolate into the batter you have made.
8. Spread the batter evenly into the pan you have prepared, and bake this until the edges of the batter just begin to become darker, and the center of the batter rises a little bit. You can also tell by sliding a toothpick into the middle, and when it comes out clean, it is ready. This will take approximately 20 to 21 minutes. Be sure that you do NOT overbake them!
9. Let them cool in the pan they cooked in for about 20 minutes. Then, carefully use the excess paper handles to take the brownies out of the pan and put them onto a wire cooling rack.
10. Make sure that they cool completely, and when they do, cut them, and they are ready to eat!

Nutrition:

- Calories: 107 kcal
- Total Fat: 10g
- Carbohydrates: 5.7g
- Protein: 2.5g

9. Apple Bread

Preparation Time: 10 Minutes
Cooking Time: 20 Minutes
Servings: 10
Ingredients:

- ½ cup of honey
- ½ tsp. of nutmeg
- ½ tsp. of salt
- 1 cup of applesauce, sweetened
- 1 tsp. of baking soda
- 1 tsp. of vanilla extract
- 2 ¼ cups of whole wheat flour
- 2 large eggs
- 2 tbsp. of vegetable oil
- 2 tsp. of baking powder
- 2 tsp. of cinnamon
- 4 cup of apples, diced

Directions:

1. Preheat oven to 375° Fahrenheit and oil a loaf pan with non-stick spray or your choice of oil.
2. Beat eggs in a mixing bowl and stir until completely smooth.
3. Add the honey, oil, applesauce, cinnamon, vanilla, nutmeg, baking powder, baking soda, and salt. Whisk until completely combined and smooth.
4. Add the flour into the bowl and whisk to combine, making sure not to over-mix. Simply stir it enough to incorporate the flour.
5. Add apples to the batter and mix once more to combine.
6. Pour the batter into the loaf pan and smooth the top with your spatula.
7. Bake for 60 minutes or until an inserted toothpick in the center comes out clean.
8. Let stand for 10 minutes, then transfer the loaf to a cooling rack to cool completely.
9. Slice into 10 pieces and serve!

Nutrition:

- Calories: 210 kcal
- Total Fat: 5g
- Carbohydrates: 41g
- Protein: 5g

10. Cinnamon and Pecan Porridge

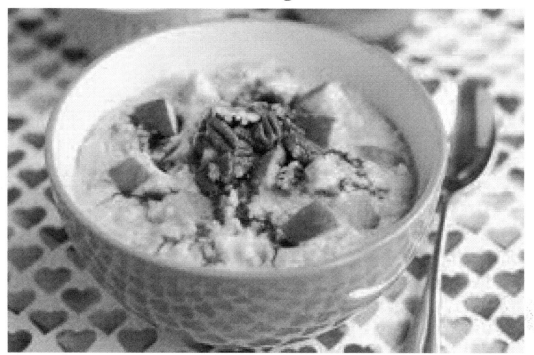

Preparation Time: 5 Minutes
Cooking Time: 10 Minutes
Servings: 2

Ingredients:

- ½ tsp. of cinnamon
- ¼ cup of pecans, chopped
- ¼ cup of unsweetened coconut, toasted
- ¼ cup of coconut milk
- ¼ cup of almond butter
- ¾ cup of unsweetened almond milk
- 1 tbsp. of extra virgin coconut oil
- 2 tbsps. of hemp seeds
- 2 tbsps. of whole chia seeds

Directions:

1. Place a small saucepan over medium heat. Combine the coconut milk, coconut oil, almond butter, and almond milk. Bring to simmer and remove from heat.
2. Add the toasted coconut (leave some for the topping), cinnamon, pecans, hemp seeds, and chia seeds. Mix the ingredients well and allow to rest for 5-10 minutes.
3. Divide between two bowls and serve.

Nutrition:

- Calories: 580 kcal
- Fat: 42g
- Fiber: 2g
- Carbs: 20g
- Protein: 7g

11. Coconut Protein Balls

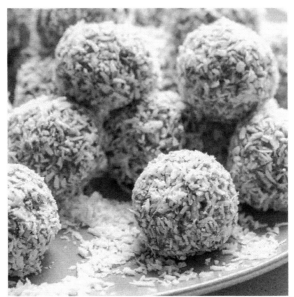

Preparation Time: 20 Minutes
Cooking Time: 0 Minutes
Servings: 27

Ingredients:

- ¼ cup of dark chocolate chips
- ½ cup of coconut flakes, unsweetened
- ½ cup of water
- 1 ½ cup of almonds, raw & unsalted
- 2 tbsp. of cocoa powder, unsweetened
- 3 cups of Medjool dates, pitted
- 4 scoops of whey protein powder, unsweetened

Directions:

1. Blend almonds in a food processor until flour is formed. Add the water and dates to the flour and continue to process until fully combined. You may need to stop intermittently to scrape down the sides of the bowl.
2. Add cocoa and protein to the processor and continue to process until well combined. You may need to stop intermittently to scrape down the sides of the bowl.
3. Pull the blade out of the processor (carefully!) and use your spatula to gather all of the dough in one place inside the processor container.
4. On a plate or in a large, shallow dish, spread the coconut flakes.
5. Scoop out a little bit of the dough at a time using a spoon, and roll it into balls, then roll each one in the coconut flakes.
6. Refrigerate for at least 30 min before enjoying.

Nutrition:

- Calories: 108 kcal
- Total Fat: 4g
- Carbohydrates: 16g
- Protein: 5g

12. Protein Bars

Preparation Time: 10 Minutes
Cooking Time: 30 Minutes
Servings: 12

Ingredients:

For the Bars:

- 1/3 cup of coconut oil
- 1/3 cup of creamy peanut butter, unsalted
- 1/3 cup of almond meal
- ½ cup milk of your choice, unsweetened
- 1 ½ cup of protein powder

For the Topping:

- 2 tbsp. of chocolate chips
- 1 tbsp. of coconut oil
- 3 tbsp. of almonds, chopped

Directions:

1. In a microwave-safe bowl, combine peanut butter, milk, and all but one tablespoon of the coconut oil. Heat for 30-second intervals, stirring in between, until completely smooth.
2. Mix almond meal and protein powder into the bowl and combine well until a crumbly dough is combined.
3. Line a baking dish with parchment paper and flatten the dough into it until an even layer is formed.
4. In a small, microwave-safe bowl, put the chocolate chips and 1 tbsp. of coconut oil and heat for 30-second intervals, while stirring in between until completely smooth.
5. Pour the mixture of chocolate over the bars and spread it evenly. Sprinkle the almonds on top and then freeze the bars for about 20 minutes, or refrigerate them for about an hour.
6. Cut into 12 evenly-shaped bars and enjoy!

Nutrition:

- Calories: 186 kcal
- Total Fat: 14g
- Carbohydrates: 7g
- Protein: 8g

13. Blueberry Muffins

Preparation Time: 5 Minutes
Cooking Time: 25 Minutes
Servings: 12

Ingredients:

- ½ tsp. of baking soda
- ¼ cup of vegetable oil
- ¼ tsp. of salt
- 1 ½ cup of blueberries, frozen
- 1 cup of applesauce, unsweetened
- 1 tsp. of vanilla extract
- 1/3 cup of honey
- 2 cups of whole wheat flour
- 1 tsp. of cinnamon
- 2 large eggs, beaten
- 2 tsp. of baking powder

Directions:

1. Preheat the oven to 350° Fahrenheit and line a muffin tin with paper liners.
2. Combine eggs, applesauce, honey, oil, vanilla extract, cinnamon, baking soda, salt and baking powder in a bowl. Whisk until completely combined, ensuring that there are no lumps of baking powder or soda.
3. Add flour to the batter and whisk until just combined.
4. Add blueberries and mix.
5. Fill the muffin tins and bake for 22-25 minutes or until a toothpick inserted into the middle of the middlemost muffin becomes clean.
6. Let cool for 30 minutes before transferring to a cooling rack to cool completely. Serve and enjoy!

Nutrition:

- Calories: 329 kcal
- Total Fat: 14g
- Carbohydrates: 40g
- Protein: 14g

14. Strawberry-Kiwi Chia Pudding

Preparation Time: 5 Minutes plus 4 Hours
Cooking Time: 0 Minutes
Servings: 2
Ingredients:

- 2 cups of unsweetened coconut milk, divided
- 3 Medjool dates, pitted
- 1 tablespoon of vanilla extract
- ½ cup of chia seeds

Toppings:

- 2 kiwis, sliced
- 4 strawberries, sliced
- 2 tablespoons of unsweetened coconut shreds
- 2 tablespoons of sliced or chopped almonds

Directions:

1. In a food processor, blend ¾ cup of coconut milk, the dates, and vanilla.

2. Pour the blended mix into a large reusable container or Mason jar.
3. Add the remaining 1¼ cups of coconut milk and the chia seeds.
4. Cover the container and shake gently or stir to mix.
5. Store in the refrigerator overnight or for at least 4 hours, until the chia seeds absorb all the milk. (Optional: stir once or twice as it is setting to avoid clumps.)
6. When ready to eat, top the pudding with the kiwi, strawberries, coconut, and almonds.
7. Store in the refrigerator for up to 5 days.

Nutrition:

- Calories: 783 kcal
- Total fat: 38g
- Carbohydrates: 79g
- Fiber: 48g
- Protein: 27g

15. Banana Churro Oatmeal

Preparation Time: 5 Minutes
Cooking Time: 10 Minutes
Servings: 2
Ingredients:

Churros:

- 1 large yellow banana, peeled, cut in half lengthwise, then cut in half widthwise
- 2 tablespoons of whole-wheat pastry flour (see Substitution Tip)
- 1/8 teaspoon of sea salt
- 2 teaspoons of oil (sunflower or melted coconut)

- 1 teaspoon of water
- Cooking oil spray (refined coconut, sunflower, or safflower)
- 1 tablespoon of coconut sugar
- ½ teaspoon of cinnamon

Oatmeal:

- ¾ cup of rolled oats
- 1½ cups of water
- Nondairy milk of your choice (optional)

Directions:

Churros:

1. Place the 4 banana pieces in a medium-size bowl and add the flour and salt.
2. Stir gently. Add the oil and water. Stir gently (ideally with a rubber spatula) until evenly mixed.
3. You may need to press some of the coating onto the banana pieces. Trust me—it's a small price to pay for what's ahead.
4. Spray the air fryer basket with the oil spray.
5. Place the banana pieces in the air fryer basket and fry for 5 minutes.
6. Remove, gently turn over, and cook for another 5 minutes (or until nicely browned).
7. In a medium bowl, add the coconut sugar and cinnamon and stir to combine. When the banana pieces are nicely browned, spray with the oil and place in the cinnamon-sugar bowl.
8. Toss gently with a spatula to coat the banana pieces with the mixture.

Oatmeal:

9. While the bananas are cooking, make your oatmeal. In a medium pot, bring the oats and water to a boil, then reduce to low heat.
10. Simmer, stirring often, until all of the water is absorbed, about 5 minutes.
11. Place the oatmeal into two bowls. If desired, pour a small amount of non-dairy milk on top (but not too much, or the banana pieces will get soggy when you add them).
12. Top your oatmeal with the coated banana pieces and serve immediately.

Nutrition:

- Calories: 266 kcal
- Total fat: 7g
- Saturated fat: 1g
- Cholesterol: 0mg
- Sodium: 120mg
- Carbohydrates: 47g
- Fiber: 6g
- Protein: 5g

16. Zucchini Muffins

Preparation Time: 5 Minutes
Cooking Time: 30 Minutes
Servings: 6

Ingredients:

- 4 scallions, chopped
- 1 tablespoon of olive oil
- 2 zucchinis, chopped
- 1 yellow bell pepper, chopped
- Salt and black pepper to the taste
- 2 tablespoons of flaxseed mixed with 3 tablespoons water
- 1 cup of almond flour
- 1 cup of almond milk
- 1 teaspoon of baking powder
- 2 tablespoons of chives, chopped

Directions:

1. Heat up a pan with the oil over medium heat, add the scallions, zucchini and the bell pepper, and sauté for 5 minutes.

2. In a bowl, combine the scallions mix with the rest of the ingredients, stir well, divide into a muffin tray and bake at 390 degrees F for 25 minutes.
3. Divide the muffins between plates and serve them for breakfast.

Nutrition:

- Calories: 258 kcal
- Fat: 21.8
- Fiber: 4.9
- Carbs: 11.9
- Protein: 6.6

17. Special Intermittent Bread

Preparation Time: 15 minutes

Cooking Time: 40 minutes

Servings: 14

Ingredients:

- 2 tsp. baking powder
- ½ cup water
- Tbsp. poppy seeds
- cups fine ground almond meal
- 5 large eggs
- ½ cup olive oil
- ½ tsp. fine Himalayan salt

Directions:

1. Preheat oven to 400°F.
2. In a bowl, combine salt, almond meal, and baking powder.
3. Drip in oil while mixing, until it forms a crumbly dough.
4. Make a little round hole in the middle of the dough and pour eggs into the middle of the dough.
5. Pour water and whisk eggs together with a mixer in the small circle until it is frothy.
6. Start making larger circles to combine the almond meal mixture with the dough until you have a smooth and thick batter.
7. Line your loaf pan with parchment paper.
8. Pour batter into the loaf pan and sprinkle poppy seeds on top.
9. Bake in the oven for 40 minutes in the center rack until firm and golden brown.
10. Cool in the oven for 30 minutes.
11. Slice and serve.

Nutrition:

- Calories: 227 kcal
- Fat: 21g
- Carb: 4g
- Protein: 7g

18. Fried Eggs with Bacon

Preparation Time: 5 minutes
Cooking Time: 10 minutes
Servings: 4

Ingredients:

- 8 medium eggs
- 5 oz. bacon
- 2 medium tomatoes
- 1 tsp chopped parsley
- 1 tbsp. ghee butter
- Salt to taste

Directions:

1. Heat the ghee butter in a skillet over medium-high heat
2. Slice the bacon and fry it until crispy for 3-4 minutes, then set aside on a paper towel
3. Meanwhile, cut the tomatoes in small cubes
4. Crack the eggs in the same skillet, add tomatoes, season with salt, and cook till the desired readiness
5. Top with the bacon and parsley. Serve hot

Nutrition:

- Carbs: 1 g
- Fat: 22 g
- Protein: 15 g
- Calories: 273 kcal

19. Chicken Sausage Breakfast Casserole

Preparation Time: 10 minutes
Cooking Time: 40 minutes
Servings: 4

Ingredients:

- 1 pound chicken sausage
- 3 big eggs
- 2 cups chopped tomatoes
- 2 cups diced zucchini
- ½ cups cheddar cheese
- ½ cup diced onion
- ½ cup plain Greek yogurt
- 1 teaspoon dried sage
- 1 teaspoon dried mustard

Directions:

1. Preheat the oven to 375°F.
2. Preheat a skillet until warm, then add sausage.
3. When nearly all the pink is gone, put the zucchini and onion.
4. Cook until the veggies are softened.
5. Move the contents of the skillet to a greased casserole dish.
6. In a separate bowl, mix eggs, yogurt, and seasonings together.
7. Lastly, mix ½ cup of cheese into eggs.
8. Pour into the casserole dish on top of the sausage and veggies.
9. Bake for at least 30 minutes until cheese has melted and starts browning.
10. Serve right away!

Nutrition:

- Calories: 487 kcal
- Protein: 19g
- Carbs: 4.8g
- Fat: 42g
- Fiber: 1.3g

20. Breakfast-Stuffed Bell Peppers

Preparation Time: 25 minutes
Cooking Time: 10 minutes
Servings: 4

Ingredients:

- 4 large yellow bell peppers
- 4 eggs
- 4 bacon strips
- 4 ounces pork breakfast sausage
- 1 cup shredded mozzarella cheese
- ½ cup diced onion
- 1 tablespoon minced garlic
- 2 teaspoons olive oil
- Salt and pepper to taste

Directions:

1. Preheat your oven to 275°F.
2. Chop the tops off the peppers and hollow out the insides.
3. Set on a baking sheet and brush the insides with a little olive oil.
4. Stick peppers in the oven.
5. Heat a skillet and cook bacon and sausage until nearly done.
6. Add onions and garlic.
7. Cook until onions have softened.
8. Take out the peppers and stuff.
9. Top with cheese and press down with a spoon, creating a little hollow.
10. Crack in an egg.
11. Turn oven up to 325°F and put the stuffed peppers in the oven for 10 minutes, or until eggs have reached the doneness you like.
12. Add salt and pepper. Serve!

Nutrition:

- Calories: 372 kcal
- Protein: 27g
- Carbs: 15g
- Fat: 24g
- Fiber: 2g

21. Small Intermittent Pies

Preparation Time: 10 minutes
Cooking Time: 30 minutes
Servings: 6

Ingredients:

- 3 eggs
- 5 bacon slices
- ½ red bell pepper
- 1 oz. leek
- ½ cup broccoli

- 1 oz. ground cheese
- ½ cup yogurt
- ¼ pack baking powder
- 1 tbsp. olive oil
- Salt, pepper, powdered garlic, and parsley to taste

4. Mix cheese with yogurt well. Then, add bacon, leek, pepper, and spices to taste.
5. Combine the two mixtures together and then pour into cupcake or muffin molds.
6. Bake for 30 minutes at 200°F.

Directions:

1. Whisk and blend the eggs with baking powder.
2. Cook the broccoli in water.
3. Cut bacon, leek, and pepper into smaller pieces to taste.

Nutrition:

- Calories: 121 kcal
- Total Fats: 2.1g
- Net Carbs: 2g
- Protein: 1.3g
- Fiber: 6g

22.   Intermittent Wraps

Preparation Time: 30 minutes
Cooking Time: 5 minutes
Servings: 6

Ingredients:

- 10 oz. turkey meat
- 3 oz. bacon
- 1 tomato
- 2 oz. mozzarella
- 2 Cabbage leaves for wrapping
- For coating:
- 1 cup mayonnaise
- 6 basil leaves
- 1 tsp. lemon juice
- 1 tsp. powdered garlic
- 1 tsp. salt
- 1 tsp. pepper

Directions:

1. Mix all ingredients listed for coating in a bowl. You should get a dense mixture.
2. Prepare bacon in a frying pan.
3. Coat cabbage leaves with the coating mixture. Pile ingredients over (turkey, tomatoes, bacon, and cheese).
4. Wrap the cabbage leaves like tortillas and serve.

Nutrition:

- Calories: 121 kcal
- Total Fats: 6.9g
- Net Carbs: 4g
- Protein: 2.4g
- Fiber: 5.6g

22.   Chicken Omelet

Preparation Time: 5 minutes
Cooking Time: 10 minutes
Servings: 2

Ingredients:

- 1 oz. rotisserie chicken, shredded
- 1 tsp. mustard
- 1 tbsp. mayonnaise
- 1 tomato, cored and chopped
- 2 bacon slices, cooked and crumbled
- 2 eggs
- 1 small avocado, pitted, peeled, and chopped
- Salt and ground black pepper, to taste

Directions:

1. Heat up a pan over medium heat, grease lightly with cooking oil.
2. Mix the eggs with some salt and pepper in a bowl and whisk.
3. Add the eggs to the pan and cook the omelet for 5 minutes.
4. Add the chicken, avocado, tomato, bacon, mayonnaise, and mustard to one half of the omelet.
5. Fold the omelet, cover the pan, cook for 5 minutes, and serve.

Nutrition:

- Calories: 400 kcal
- Total Fats: 32g
- Net Carbs: 4g
- Protein: 25g
- Fiber: 6g

23.   Coconut Pancakes

Preparation Time: 10 minutes

Cooking Time: 10 minutes

Servings: 2

Ingredients:

- 4 tablespoons coconut flour
- 3 ounces coconut milk
- 2 eggs

- 1 tablespoon melted coconut oil
- Pinch salt
- ½ teaspoon baking powder
- 1 ounce coconut oil (or butter) for frying
- 1 teaspoon erythritol (optional)

Directions:

1. If you want fluffy pancakes, separate the egg whites and whisk them with a

pinch of salt until stiff peaks form. If you don't have enough time, skip this step.

2. In another bowl, mix the egg yolks (wholes eggs if you skip the first step), coconut milk, and melted coconut oil (it has to be at room temperature so it doesn't burn egg yolks).

3. Add in coconut flour, baking powder, and sweetener (if used) and mix well until smooth.

4. Slowly transfer the egg whites to the batter. Set aside for 3-5 minutes.

5. Preheat an oiled (or buttered) skillet at medium-low heat. Fry pancakes for 2-4 minutes on both sides until golden brown. Flip them gently.

6. Serve coconut pancakes with sour cream, whipped cream, or your favorite intermittent-friendly toppings (do not forget about carbs in berries and cream).

Nutrition:

- Calories: 328 kcal
- Total Carbs: 9g
- Fiber: 5g
- Net Carbs: 4g
- Fat: 28g
- Protein: 9g

Chapter 13:   Healthy Recipes - Lunch

24.   Ground Beef and Cauliflower Hash

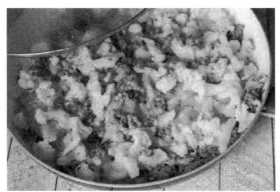

Preparation Time: 10 Minutes
Cooking Time: 25 Minutes
Servings: 6

Ingredients:

- 1 (16-ounce) bag of frozen cauliflower florets, defrosted and drained
- 1 pound of lean grass-fed ground beef
- 2 cups of shredded cheddar cheese
- 1 teaspoon of garlic powder
- ½ teaspoon of fine sea salt
- ½ teaspoon of freshly cracked black pepper

Directions:

1. In a large skillet over medium-high heat, add the ground beef and cook until brown. Drain the excess grease.

2. Add the cauliflower florets, garlic powder, fine sea salt and freshly cracked black pepper. Cook until the cauliflower is tender, stirring occasionally.
3. Add the shredded cheddar cheese to the cauliflower and ground beef mixture.
4. Remove from the heat and cover with a lid. Allow the steam to melt the cheese.
5. Serve and enjoy!

Nutrition:

- Calories: 311 kcal
- Fat: 7g
- Fiber: 2g
- Carbs: 5g
- Protein: 33g

25.   Cheesy Taco Skillet

Preparation Time: 10 Minutes
Cooking Time: 20 Minutes
Servings: 4

Ingredients:

- 1 pound of lean grass-fed ground beef
- 1 large yellow or white onions, finely chopped
- 2 medium-sized bell peppers, finely chopped
- 1 (12-ounce) can of diced tomatoes with green chilis
- 2 large zucchinis, finely chopped
- 2 tablespoons of taco seasoning
- 3 cups of fresh baby kale or fresh spinach
- 1 ½ cups of shredded cheddar cheese OR shredded jack cheese

Directions:

1. In a large nonstick skillet, add the ground beef and cook until lightly brown. Drain the excess grease.
2. Add the chopped onions, chopped bell peppers, diced tomatoes with green chilis, zucchini and taco seasoning. Cook for 5 minutes, stirring occasionally.
3. Add the fresh baby kale or spinach. Cook until wilted.
4. Cover with 1 ½ cups of shredded cheddar cheese and cover with a lid.
5. Once the cheese has melted, serve and enjoy!

Nutrition:

- Calories: 287 kcal
- Fat: 8g
- Fiber: 2g
- Carbs: 12g
- Protein 28g

26.   Zoodle Soup with Italian Meatballs

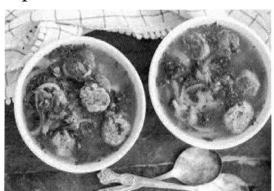

Preparation Time: 20 Minutes
Cooking Time: 6 Hours and 25 Minutes
Servings: 12

Ingredients:

- 1 ½ pound of lean grass-fed beef
- 4 cups of homemade low-sodium beef stock
- 1 medium-sized zucchini, spiralized
- 2 celery ribs, finely chopped
- 1 small yellow or white onion, finely chopped
- 1 medium carrot, chopped
- 1 medium tomato, finely chopped
- 1 tablespoon of extra-virgin olive oil.
- ½ cup of shredded parmesan cheese
- 1 large egg
- 4 tablespoons of fresh parsley, finely chopped
- 1 teaspoon of fine sea salt
- ½ teaspoon of garlic powder
- 1 teaspoon of onion powder
- 1 teaspoon of Italian seasoning
- 1 teaspoon of dried oregano
- ½ teaspoon of freshly cracked black pepper

Directions:

1. Add the 4 cups of beef stock, spiralized zucchini, chopped celery, chopped onions, chopped carrot, and chopped tomatoes inside a slow cooker.
2. In a large bowl, add the ground beef, shredded parmesan cheese, garlic powder, fine sea salt, egg, fresh parsley, onion powder, Italian seasoning, dried oregano and freshly cracked black pepper. Stir until well incorporated.
3. Form the ground beef mixture into meatballs.
4. In a large non-stick skillet over medium-high heat add the olive oil, working in batches, add the meatballs and cook until brown.
5. Add the meatballs to the slow cooker and cover with a lid.
6. Cook on "Low" for 6 hours. Serve and enjoy!

Nutrition:

- Calories: 129 kcal
- Fat: 12g
- Fiber: 2g
- Carbs: 20g
- Protein: 16g

27. Mini Thai Lamb Salad Bites

Preparation Time: 10 Minutes
Cooking Time: 8 Minutes
Servings: 15

Ingredients:

- 1 large cucumber, cut into 0.39-inch-thick diagonal rounds
- 0.55 lb. (250g) of Lamb Blackstrap
- ¾ cup of cherry Tomatoes, quartered
- 1/3 cup of fresh mint, loosely packed
- 1/3 cup of fresh coriander, loosely packed
- ¼ of a small red onion, finely diced
- 1 tsp. of fish sauce
- Juice of 1 lime
- Coconut oil

Directions:

1. Place pan over medium heat and heat oil. Cook the lamb for 4 minutes on each side. Remove from heat and let it rest.
2. In a mixing bowl, toss the onions, tomatoes, mint, coriander, fish sauce, and lime juice.
3. Cut the lamb into thin strips and add it to the salad bowl. Toss to combine.
4. Spoon ample amount of mixture on each cucumber cut. Chill and serve.

Nutrition:

- Calories: 58 kcal
- Fat: 2g
- Fiber: 2g
- Carbs: 20g
- Protein: 5g

28.   Smoked Salmon & Avocado Stacks

Preparation Time: 15 Minutes
Cooking Time: 0 Minutes
Servings: 6

Ingredients:

- ½ lb. of smoked salmon, finely diced
- 1 ripe avocado, seed removed and diced
- 1 tbsp. of chives, chopped
- Fresh or dried dill leaves
- 3 tsps. of fresh lemon juice
- Black pepper, cracked

Directions:

1. Mix salmon, chives, and a teaspoon of lemon juice in a small mixing bowl.

2. In another mixing bowl, toss the avocado, remaining lemon juice, and pepper.
3. Using a presentation ring, arrange the stacks on the serving plates. Arrange the avocado at the bottom and top it with the salmon mixture and gently press. Remove the mold and garnish the stack with dill leaves. Serve chilled.

Nutrition:

- Calories: 106 kcal
- Fat: 12g
- Fiber: 2g
- Carbs: 20g
- Protein: 5g

29.   Sesame-Seared Salmon

Preparation Time: 5 Minutes
Cooking Time: 10 Minutes
Servings: 4

Ingredients:

- 4 wild salmon fillets (about 1lb.)
- 1½ tbsps. of sesame seeds
- 2 tbsps. of toasted sesame oil
- 1½ tbsps. of avocado oil
- 1 tsp. of sea salt

Directions:

1. Using a paper towel or a clean kitchen towel, pat the fillets to dry. Brush each with a tablespoon of sesame oil and season with a half teaspoon of salt.

2. Place a large skillet over medium-high heat and drizzle with avocado oil. Once the oil is hot, add the salmon fillets with the flesh side down. Cook for about 3 minutes and flip. Cook the skin side for an additional 3-4 minutes, without overcooking it.
3. Remove the pan from the heat and brush with the remaining sesame oil. Season with the remaining salt and sprinkle with sesame seeds. Best served with green salad.

Nutrition:

- Calories: 198 kcal
- Fat: 12g
- Fiber: 2g
- Carbs: 20g
- Protein: 5g

30. Spring Ramen Bowl

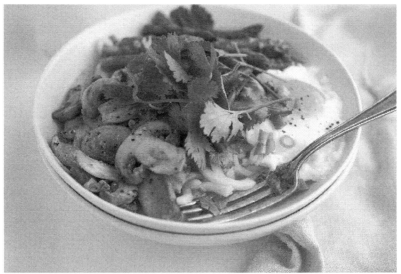

Preparation Time: 10 Minutes
Cooking Time: 20 Minutes
Servings: 6
Ingredients:

- 3.53 oz. (100g) of soba noodles
- 4 eggs
- 1 medium zucchini, julienned or grated
- 4 cups of chicken stock
- 2 cups of watercress
- ½ cup of snap peas
- 1 cup of mushrooms, finely sliced
- 1 leek (white part only), finely sliced
- 2 garlic cloves, minced
- 1 long red chili, seeded and finely chopped
- 1.6-inch ginger, minced
- 1 tsp. of sesame oil
- 2 nori sheets, crumbled
- 1 lemon, cut into wedges
- 1 tbsp. of olive oil

Directions:

1. To boil the eggs, fill a saucepan with enough water to cover the eggs and set it over medium heat. Bring water to a gentle boil. Add the eggs and cook for 7 minutes. Drain and transfer the eggs into cold water. Set aside.
2. Place a medium-sized saucepan over medium-low heat. Heat the olive oil and sauté the garlic, ginger, leek, and chili for 5 minutes. Add the stock, noodles, and sesame oil. Cook for another 8 minutes or until noodles are cooked according to your desired doneness. In the last minute, add the zucchini, mushroom, and watercress.
3. Divide the ramen between four bowls and top them with nori. Serve with the eggs and lemon wedges.

Nutrition:

- Calories: 340 kcal
- Fat: 23g
- Fiber: 2g
- Carbs: 8g
- Protein: 28g

31. Homemade Turkey Burger and Relish

Preparation Time: 10 Minutes
Cooking Time: 20 Minutes
Servings: 4

Ingredients:

- 2lb ground of turkey, made into four patties
- 1 onion, finely chopped
- 1 red bell pepper, chopped up finely
- 3 cups of red cabbage, chopped or shredded
- 1 tbsp. of olive oil
- 0.25 cup of balsamic vinegar
- 0.25 tsp. of garlic salt
- 4 lettuce leaves, large if possible

Directions:

1. Take a large skillet pan and place over a medium heat.
2. Add the olive oil and allow it to reach temperature.
3. Add the onion, red cabbage and pepper to the pan and cook until everything has softened
4. Now add the balsamic vinegar and the garlic salt and combine everything together, letting it simmer for a few minutes until the contents have caramelized from the vinegar.
5. Remove the contents of the pan and set them aside to cool.
6. Take your turkey patties and season them with salt and pepper.
7. Cook your patties for around 4 minutes on each side in either a pan or under the grill.
8. Once cooked, transfer each patty onto a lettuce leaf and add some of the relishes on top.

Nutrition:

- Calories: 198 kcal
- Fat: 12g
- Fiber: 2g
- Carbs: 20g
- Protein: 5g

32.　Chicken Cobb Salad, With a BBQ Twist

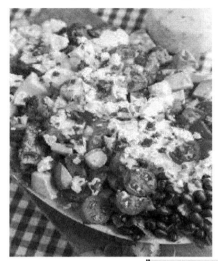

Preparation Time: 10 Minutes
Cooking Time: 25 Minutes
Servings: 4

Ingredients:

- 3oz chicken breast, no bones, and no skin
- 2 tbsp. of BBQ sauce
- 2 slices of bacon, chopped into small pieces
- 1.5 cups of romaine lettuce, chopped
- 0.25 cups of cherry tomatoes, chopped
- 0.25 of avocado, chopped
- 1 boiled egg, chopped

Directions:

1. Preheat your oven to 350C.
2. Take the chicken and brush it with 1 tbsp of the BBQ sauce.
3. Take a baking dish and spray with a little cooking spray.
4. Place the chicken inside the baking dish and place into the oven for 25 minutes, or until the chicken is completely cooked through.
5. Whilst the chicken is cooking, cook your bacon according to your preference and chop up once cooked.
6. Take a serving bowl and place your romaine lettuce inside, arranging carefully.
7. Add the chicken and bacon once cooked, as well as the egg, tomatoes, and the avocado.
8. Drizzle the rest of the BBQ sauce over the top and enjoy whilst still warm.

Nutrition:

- Calories: 250 kcal
- Fat: 8g
- Fiber: 2g
- Carbs: 8g
- Protein: 17g

33. Hearty Quinoa and Carrot Soup

Preparation Time: 10 Minutes
Cooking Time: 50 Minutes
Servings: 4

Ingredients:

- 1 tbsp. of coconut oil
- 1 medium onion, chopped
- 1 small shallot, chopped very finely
- 1 tsp. of garlic, minced
- 1 tsp. of thyme, fresh is best in this case
- 3 sage leaves, chopped. Again, go for fresh if you can
- 1 tsp. of cumin
- 0.25 tsp. of turmeric
- A little black pepper, according to your preferences
- 1lb of carrots, chopped
- 0.5lb of parsnips, chopped
- 0.25 cup of quinoa, uncooked, and ensure it is rinsed out and drained thoroughly
- 5 cups of broth, a vegetable broth is best, or you can simply use water

Directions:

1. For this recipe, you will need a large saucepan or stockpot.
2. Add the coconut oil and place over a medium heat.
3. Once hot, add the garlic, onion, and the shallot, and cook for around 6 minutes.
4. Add the cumin, turmeric, thyme and the sage, with the pepper, and combine well.
5. Now, add the parsnips and the carrots and stir once more.
6. Add the quinoa and stir again.
7. Add the broth or the water and allow the mixture to boil.
8. Once the pan boils, turn the heat down to a simmer.
9. Cook for 30-40 minutes, until everything is soft and cooked through.
10. Take the pan from the heat and place it aside for around 5 minutes, until it has cooked down.
11. You will now need an immersion or hand blender, so you can blend up the cup until it is smooth.
12. Serve while still warm.

Nutrition:

- Calories: 185 kcal
- Fat: 12g
- Fiber: 2g
- Carbs: 4g
- Protein: 11g

34. Warming Lamb Stew

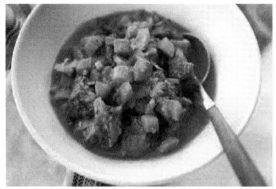

Preparation Time: 15 Minutes
Cooking Time: 1 Hour and 20 Minutes
Servings: 7

Ingredients:

- 2 tsp of olive oil, extra virgin is best
- 1lb lamb, make sure it is as lean as you can get it, and cut into cubes
- A little salt
- A little pepper
- 1 large onion, chopped
- 1 celery stalk, chopped
- 2 garlic cloves, chopped
- 2 carrots, cut into small pieces
- 1.5 tsp. of oregano
- 2 cups of broth, chicken broth works best here but you can use vegetable also
- 0.25 cup of red wine, the dry version works well
- 1x15oz can of tomato sauce, the smoother the better
- 1 tsp. of zest from a lemon
- 0.5 tsp of cinnamon
- 1 sweet potato, chopped
- 1 lemon, chopped

Directions:

1. You will need a Dutch oven for this recipe, and you need to add the oil and set to a medium-high heat.
2. Once heated up, add the meat and add a little salt and pepper to your taste.
3. Sear the lamb on both sides.
4. Now, add the celery and the onion and cook for around 4 minutes, until soft.
5. Add the garlic and cook for half a minute.
6. Add the oregano and combine well, and then add the carrots, stirring all the while for another half a minute.
7. Add the wine, the broth, the tomato sauce, the lemon zest, and the cinnamon and combine everything well.
8. Next, add the sweet potato and the lemon and combine once more.
9. Allow the mixture to reach the boiling point and then turn the heat down to a lower temperature, covering over and allowing to simmer.
10. Cook until the vegetables are soft, and the lamb is totally cooked, for between 80-90 minutes.
11. You may need to add more salt and pepper, according to your personal preferences.

Nutrition:

- Calories: 280 kcal
- Fat: 8g
- Fiber: 2g
- Carbs: 7g
- Protein: 8g

35.   Spicy Chicken Masala

Preparation Time: 10 Minutes
Cooking Time: 20 Minutes
Servings: 4

Ingredients:

- 4 chicken cutlets, pounded until they are quite thin
- A little salt to taste
- 1 egg, beaten
- 0.5 cup of whole-wheat flour, plus another 1.5 tbsp
- 2 x 8oz packs of button mushrooms, sliced
- 4 cloves of garlic, minced
- 0.5 cup of Marsala wine, the dry version works best
- 1 cup of chicken broth, low fat is best
- 0.25 cup of Greek yogurt
- A little black pepper
- Cheese for topping if you want to

Directions:

1. You will need two non-stick pans for this recipe, and they both need to be placed over a medium-low heat.
2. Season your chicken with a little salt and wait for the pans to heat up, spraying with a little cooking oil.
3. In a small mixing bowl, add the beaten egg and the half cup of whole-wheat flour and mix together.
4. Dip the chicken into the mixture and cover completely, before placing it into the pans, two in each.
5. Cook the chicken for about 4 minutes on each side and then.
6. Place the chicken onto a plate and keep warm with aluminum foil.
7. Clean the pans out and turn the heat up, adding a little more spray to the pans.
8. Place one package of mushrooms into each pan and cook for around 3 minutes.
9. Now, place all the mushrooms in one pan and add the garlic and a little salt.
10. Turn the heat down and cook for one more minute.
11. Add the rest of the whole-wheat flour to the mixture, along with the wine and the broth, mixing everything well.
12. Allow the mixture to simmer, for around 3 minutes.
13. Take the pan off the heat and add the yogurt and a little more salt and pepper, stirring well.
14. Remove the foil from the chicken and place on a serving plate, pouring the Marsala sauce over the top.
15. Add a little cheese to melt on top if you like.

Nutrition:

- Calories: 340 kcal
- Fat: 15g
- Fiber: 2g
- Carbs: 18g
- Protein: 30g

36. Quick Ratatouille

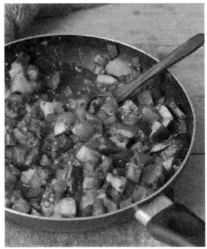

Preparation Time: 10 Minutes
Cooking Time: 12 Minutes
Servings: 4

Ingredients:

- 2 onions, sliced
- 4 cloves of garlic, chopped very finely
- 0.5 cup of olive oil
- 1 green pepper, cut into small pieces
- 1 red pepper, cut into small pieces
- 1 aubergine (eggplant), cut into cubes
- 4 zucchinis, cubed
- 8 tomatoes, seeded and chopped
- 1.5 tsp. of salt
- A little black pepper

Directions:

1. You will need a large and deep-frying pan or saucepan.
2. Add the oil and allow to reach a medium-high heat.
3. Add the onions and the garlic and cook for a few minutes, until the onions are clear.
4. Add the peppers, zucchini, and the aborigine (eggplant) and mix.
5. Turn the heat down and cover the pan, allowing it to simmer for around 10 minutes.
6. Add the salt and pepper, as well as the tomatoes, and stir well, covering the pan once more and allowing it to continue cooking for another 10 minutes.
7. Take the lid off the pan and stir the mixture, allowing it to reduce.
8. Add a little salt and pepper and serve while still warm. The mixture is done when it is blended well, but isn't particularly "wet."

Nutrition:

- Calories: 270 kcal
- Fat: 8g
- Fiber: 2g
- Carbs: 8g
- Protein: 6g

37. Intermittent Chicken Enchaladas

Preparation Time: 10 minutes

Cooking Time: 25 minutes

Servings: 6

Ingredients:

- 2 cups gluten-free enchilada sauce

Chicken:

- 1 tablespoon Avocado oil
- 4 garlic cloves, minced
- 3 cups shredded chicken, cooked
- ¼ cup chicken broth
- ¼ cup fresh cilantro, chopped

Assembly:

- Coconut tortillas
- ¾ cup Colby jack cheese, shredded
- ¼ cup green onions, chopped

Direction:

1. Warm oil at medium to high heat in a large pan. Add the chopped garlic and cook until fragrant for about a minute.
2. Add rice, 1 cup of enchilada sauce (half the total), chicken, and coriander. Simmer for 5 minutes.
3. In the meantime, heat the oven to 375°F. Grease a 9x13" baking dish.
4. In the middle of each tortilla, place ¼ cup of the chicken mixture. Roll up and place seam side down in the baking dish.
5. Pour the remaining cup of enchilada sauce over the enchiladas. Sprinkle with shredded cheese.
6. Bake for 10 to 12 minutes. Sprinkle with green onions.

Nutrition:

- Calories: 349 kcal
- Fat: 19g
- Net Carbs: 9g
- Protein: 31g

38.   Pesto Pork Chops

Preparation Time: 20 minutes

Cooking Time: 22 minutes

Servings: 3

Ingredients:

- 3(3-ounce) top-flood pork chops, boneless, fat
- 8 table spoons Herb Pesto
- ½ cup bread crumbs
- 1 table spoon olive oil

Directions:

1. Preheat the oven to 360°F. Cover a foil baker's sheet; set aside.
2. Rub 1 tablespoon of pesto evenly across each pork chop on both sides.
3. Lightly dredge every pork chop in the breadcrumbs.
4. Heat the oil in a medium-high heat large skillet. Brown the pork chops for about 6 minutes on each side.
5. Place the pork chops on the baking sheet. Bake until the pork reaches 136°F in the center for about 10 minutes.

Nutrition:

- Fat: 8 g
- Carbohydrates: 10 g
- Phosphorus: 188 mg
- Potassium: 220 mg
- Sodium: 138 mg
- Protein: 23 g

39.   Sausage and Cauliflower Rice

Preparation time: 5 minutes
Cooking time: 20 minutes;
Servings: 2

Ingredients:

- 7 oz grated cauliflower
- 3 oz sausage
- 1 green onion, sliced
- ½ tsp garlic powder
- 2 tbsp avocado oil
- 1/3 tsp salt
- ¼ tsp ground black pepper
- 6 tbsp water

Directions:

1. Take a medium skillet pan, place it over medium heat, add 1 tablespoon of oil and when hot, add sausage and cook for 4 to 5 minutes until nicely browned.
2. Switch heat to medium-low level, pour in 4 tablespoons of water and then simmer for 5 to 7 minutes until sausage has thoroughly cooked.
3. Transfer sausage to a bowl, wipe clean the pan, then return it over medium heat, add oil and when hot, add cauliflower rice and green onion and

sprinkle with garlic powder, salt, and black pepper.
4. Stir until mixed, drizzle with 2 tablespoons of water, and cook for 5 minutes until softened.
5. Add the sausage, stir until mixed, cook for 1 minute until hot and then serve.

Nutrition:
- Calories: 333 kcal
- Fats: 31.3 g
- Protein: 9.1 g
- Net Carb: 0.8 g
- Fiber: 2.5 g

40. Double Cheese Meatloaf

Preparation time: 10 minutes
Cooking time: 25 minutes
Servings: 2

Ingredients:
- 2 bacon slices, chopped, cooked
- 6 oz. sausage
- 2 tbsp. grated mozzarella cheese
- 2 tbsp. grated cheddar cheese
- 1/3 tsp. salt
- ¼ tsp. ground black pepper
- 1 tsp. dried parsley
- 2 tbsp. marinara sauce
- 1 egg

Directions:
1. Turn on the oven, then set it to 375°F and let it preheat.
2. Meanwhile, take a medium bowl, place all the ingredients in it except for marinara, and stir until well combined.
3. Spoon the mixture into a mini loaf pan, top with marinara, and then bake for 20 to 25 minutes until cooked through and done.
4. When done, let meatloaf cool for 5 minutes, then cut it into slices and then serve.

Nutrition:
- Calories: 578 kcal
- Fats: 50.6 g
- Protein: 27.4 g
- Net Carb: 2.6 g
- Fiber: 0.3 g

41. Beef with Cabbage Noodles

Preparation time: 5 minutes
Cooking time: 18 minutes
Servings: 2

Ingredients:
- 4 oz. ground beef
- 1 cup chopped cabbage
- 4 oz. tomato sauce
- ½ tsp. minced garlic
- ½ cup of water

- ½ tbsp.. coconut oil
- ½ tsp. salt
- ¼ tsp. Italian seasoning
- 1/8 tsp. dried basil

Directions:

1. Take a skillet pan, place it over medium heat, add oil and when hot, add beef and cook for 5 minutes until nicely browned.
2. Meanwhile, prepare the cabbage and for it, slice the cabbage into thin shred.
3. When the beef has cooked, add garlic, season with salt, basil, and Italian seasoning, stir well and continue cooking for 3 minutes until beef has thoroughly cooked.
4. Pour in tomato sauce and water, stir well, and bring the mixture to boil.

5. Then reduce heat to medium-low level, add cabbage, stir well until well mixed, and simmer for 3 to 5 minutes until cabbage is softened, covering the pan.
6. Uncover the pan and continue simmering the beef until most of the cooking liquid has evaporated.
7. Serve.

Nutrition:

- Calories: 188.5 kcal
- Fats: 12.5 g
- Protein: 15.5 g
- Net Carb: 2.5 g
- Fiber: 1 g

42. Roast Beef and Mozzarella Plate

Preparation time: 5 minutes
Cooking time: 0 minutes
Servings: 2

Ingredients:

- 4 slices of roast beef
- ½ ounce chopped lettuce
- 1 avocado, pitted
- 2 oz. mozzarella cheese, cubed
- ½ cup mayonnaise
- ¼ tsp. salt
- 1/8 tsp. ground black pepper
- 2 tbsp. avocado oil

Directions:

1. Scoop out the flesh from avocado and divide it evenly between two plates.
2. Add slices of roast beef, lettuce, and cheese and then sprinkle with salt and black pepper.
3. Serve with avocado oil and mayonnaise.

Nutrition:

- Calories: 267.7 kcal
- Fats: 24.5 g
- Protein: 9.5 g
- Net Carb: 1.5 g
- Fiber: 2 g

43.   Sprouts Stir-fry with Kale, Broccoli, and Beef

Preparation time: 5 minutes
Cooking time: 8 minutes
Servings: 2

Ingredients:

- 3 slices of beef roast, chopped
- 2 oz. Brussels sprouts, halved
- 4 oz. broccoli florets
- 3 oz. kale
- 1 ½ tbsp. butter, unsalted
- 1/8 tsp. red pepper flakes

Seasoning:
- ¼ tsp. garlic powder
- ¼ tsp. salt
- 1/8 tsp. ground black pepper

Directions:

1. Take a medium skillet pan, place it over medium heat, add ¾ tablespoon butter and when it melts, add broccoli florets, sprouts, and red pepper flakes, sprinkle with garlic powder, and cook for 2 minutes.
2. Season vegetables with salt and ground black pepper, add chopped beef, stir until mixed, and continue cooking for 3 minutes until browned on one side.
3. Then add kale along with remaining butter, flip the vegetables and cook for 2 minutes until kale leaves wilted.
4. Serve.

Nutrition:

- Calories: 125 kcal
- Fats: 9.4 g
- Protein: 4.8 g
- Net Carb: 1.7 g
- Fiber: 2.6 g

44.   Fennel & Figs Lamb

Preparation Time: 10 minutes

Cooking Time: 40 minutes

Servings: 2

Ingredients:

- 6 ounces lamb racks
- 2 fennel bulbs, sliced
- Salt to taste
- Pepper to taste
- 1 tablespoon olive oil
- 2 figs, cut in half
- 1/8 cup apple cider vinegar
- ½ tablespoon swerve

Directions:

1. Take a bowl and add fennel, figs, vinegar, swerve, oil, and toss. Transfer to a baking dish. Season with salt and pepper.
2. Bake it for 15 minutes at 400°F.
3. Season lamb with salt and pepper, and transfer to a heated pan over medium-high heat. Cook for a few minutes. Add lamb to

the baking dish with fennel and bake for 20 minutes. Divide between plates and serve. Enjoy!

Nutrition:

- Calories: 230 kcal
- Fat: 3g
- Carbohydrates: 5g
- Protein: 10g
- Fiber: 2g
- Net Carbohydrates: 3g

Chapter 13: Healthy Recipes - Dinner

45. Cajun Chicken with Buckwheat Crust

Preparation Time: 10 Minutes
Cooking Time: 20 Minutes
Servings: 4

Ingredients:

- 0.25 cup of buckwheat flour
- 2 tbsp. of paprika powder, the sweet version is the best for this recipe
- 1 tsp. of turmeric powder
- 1 tsp. of cumin powder
- 1 tsp. of coriander powder
- A little salt
- A little pepper
- 0.5 tsp. of cinnamon powder
- A little coconut oil for cooking
- 4 chicken breasts, but you can use thighs if you prefer
- 1 red chili pepper, chopped very finely (be careful to wash your hands!)
- A few almonds, chopped very finely

Directions:

1. Take a mixing bowl and mix the flour and the powders
2. Take your chicken and coat evenly with the mixture
3. Take a large frying pan and add the coconut oil, allowing it to heat up over a medium to low heat
4. Place the chicken in the pan and cook on both sides until completely cooked through
5. Once cooked, transfer to a serving plate and serve with the finely chopped chili and the almonds
6. Add a little salt and pepper according to your personal preference

Nutrition:

- Calories: 345 kcal
- Fat: 8g
- Fiber: 2g
- Carbs: 8g
- Protein: 45g

46. Healthy Mushroom and Arugula Pizza

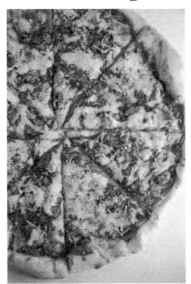

Preparation Time: 10 Minutes
Cooking Time: 20 Minutes
Servings: 4

Ingredients:

- Enough cornmeal to coat a 14" pizza pan
- 0.5lb of wild mushrooms. You can go for a mix if you want to, including chanterelles, and porcini as some of the most flavorsome
- 2 tbsp. of olive oil
- A little salt and pepper
- 2 cups of arugula leaves, chopped roughly
- 1.5 tsp. of lemon juice, go for fresh for the best taste
- 1 cup of grated cheese, Gruyere is ideal for this pizza
- 1 pack of pizza dough

Directions:

1. Preheat your oven to 260F
2. Take a 14" pizza pan and cover the base with the cornmeal evenly
3. Take an oven-proof dish and add 1 tbsp of the oil and the mushrooms
4. Add a little salt and pepper and stir everything to ensure it is evenly coated
5. Place in the oven for 10 minutes and then set aside
6. Take a mixing bowl and combine the lemon juice, the rest of the oil and the arugula, seasoning with salt and pepper
7. Next, make your pizza dough according to directions and brush the edge with a little extra olive oil
8. Add the cheese on top of the dough evenly
9. Add the mushrooms, but make sure you leave around 2 inches towards the edge
10. Place in the oven for around 10 minutes
11. Once cooked, place it to one side to cool for a couple of minutes
12. Cut into slices and place some of the arugula mixture on top

Nutrition:

- Calories: 354 kcal
- Fat: 14g
- Fiber: 2g
- Carbs: 16g
- Protein: 26g

47. Easy Mexican Casserole

Preparation Time: 10 Minutes
Cooking Time: 45 Minutes
Servings: 3

Ingredients:

- 1 cauliflower head
- 0.5 of onion, chopped
- 1 red bell pepper, chopped
- 1 green pepper, chopped
- 1 jalapeño pepper, chopped
- 1 tsp. of cumin
- 1 tsp. of chili powder
- 8 tomatoes, cherry work best, cut into halves
- 1.5 cups of cheese, shredded

Directions:

1. Preheat your oven to 240C
2. Take a large skillet pan and heat up over medium heat, with little olive oil
3. Add the onions, chili powder, cumin, and the peppers and combine well, cooking for around 2 minutes
4. Remove from the heat and place to one side
5. Crumble the cauliflower up into small pieces and place in the microwave for around 3 minutes
6. Once finished, add the tomatoes and 1 cup of cheese and combine well
7. Add to the pepper mixture and combine once more
8. Take a medium baking dish and coat with cooking spray
9. Place the ingredients into the dish and spread evenly
10. Add the rest of the cheese and cook for half an hour
11. Allow to cool a little before slicing up and serving

Nutrition:

- Calories: 354 kcal
- Fat: 14g
- Fiber: 2g
- Carbs: 16g
- Protein: 26g

48. Southwest Chicken Salad

Preparation Time: 15 Minutes
Cooking Time: 15 Minutes
Servings: 8

Ingredients:

- ¼ cup of extra virgin olive oil
- ¼ cup of red onion, finely chopped
- 1 cup of corn, drained
- 1 can of low-sodium black beans, rinsed & drained
- 1 jalapeño, seeded & minced
- 1 tsp. of chili powder
- 1 tsp. of cumin
- 1 tsp. of garlic powder
- 1 tsp. of onion powder
- 2 bell peppers, diced
- 2 lb. of limes, juiced
- 2 lb. of chicken thighs, cooked and diced
- 2 tbsp. of cilantro, finely chopped
- 3 cups of quinoa, cooked
- Sea salt and black pepper, to taste

Directions:

1. In a small bowl, mix chili powder, lime juice, onion powder, garlic powder, cumin, and cilantro. Mix thoroughly and set aside.
2. In a large mixing bowl, combine all other ingredients and toss until thoroughly combined.
3. Drizzle seasoning mixture over the salad and toss to coat completely.
4. Cover and refrigerate for 30 minutes before serving.

Nutrition:

- Calories: 217 kcal,
- Total Fat: 9g,
- Carbohydrates: 30g,
- Protein: 7g

49. Stuffed Portobello Mushrooms

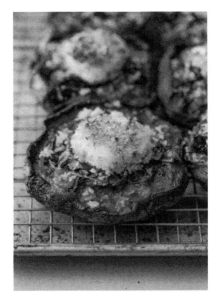

Preparation Time: 10 Minutes
Cooking Time: 20 Minutes

Servings: 4

Ingredients:

- 8 portobello mushrooms, the large ones are best
- 6-oz kale, the fresher the better
- 8 slices of cheese, go for the one you like more
- 2 tbsp. of olive oil, extra virgin is best here also

Directions:

1. Preheat your oven to 250C
2. Take a baking sheet and cover it with parchment paper
3. Place the mushrooms onto the tray, with the "cup" facing upwards
4. Drizzle a little of the olive oil over the top of the mushrooms and place in the oven for around 10 minutes
5. Once cooked, add a slice of cheese to each mushroom and a little of the kale
6. Place back in the oven for another 3 minutes; the mushrooms are cooked when the cheese is melted and bubbling
7. Allow cooling a little before serving

Nutrition:

- Calories: 320 kcal
- Fat: 8g
- Fiber: 2g
- Carbs: 0g
- Protein: 34g

50. Quinoa and Turkey Stuffed Peppers

Preparation Time: 5 Minutes
Cooking Time: 55 Minutes
Servings: 7

Ingredients:

- 2 tbsp. of extra virgin olive oil
- 1 onion, red is best, diced
- 3 cloves of garlic
- 1 chipotle pepper, the larger the better, minced up
- 1-lb lean turkey mince
- 1 tsp. of paprika, go for smoked if you can
- 1 tsp. of cumin
- 0.5 tsp. of salt
- 025 tsp. of black pepper
- 15oz fire-roasted tomatoes, cut into small pieces
- 0.75 cup of drained black beans
- 0.75 cup of corn, frozen works well here
- 0.25 cup of cilantro, fresh if possible, diced
- 0.5 cup of quinoa, dried
- 7 bell peppers, with the top, cut off and deseeded
- 0.75 cup of cheese, shredded

Directions:

1. Preheat your oven to 240C
2. Take a saucepan and add a cup of water, allowing it to boil
3. Once the water boils, add the quinoa and cover over, bringing it to the boil once more
4. Reduce the quinoa down to a simmer, for around 12 minutes, before fluffing it up and putting it to one side
5. Take a large frying pan and add a little oil, setting over a medium-high heat
6. Add the diced onions and cook for around 3 minutes
7. Add the chipotle pepper and the garlic and cook for another minute
8. Add the paprika, salt, pepper, cumin, and the tomatoes, the cilantro, corn, and the beans, and mix everything together
9. Cook for around 5 minutes, until all the liquid has disappeared
10. Toss the turkey mince with the quinoa and add to the other ingredients, mixing together well
11. Take a large baking dish and spray with a little cooking oil
12. Place the peppers into the dish, making sure they won't fall over
13. Add the turkey mixture to the inside of each pepper
14. Place in the oven for 40 minutes
15. Add a little of the shredded cheese to the top of each pepper and place back in the oven for another one minute
16. Once cooked, add the cilantro and serve

Nutrition:

- Calories: 415 kcal
- Fat: 35g
- Fiber: 2g
- Carbs: 8g
- Protein: 20g

51. Parmesan Roasted Cabbage

Preparation Time: 5 minutes
Cooking Time: 20 minutes
Servings: 4

Ingredients:

- 1 large head of green cabbage
- 4 tbsp. melted butter
- 1 tsp. garlic powder
- Salt and black pepper to taste
- 1 cup grated Parmesan cheese
- Grated Parmesan cheese for topping
- 1 tbsp. chopped parsley to garnish

Directions:

1. Set the oven to 400°F, line a baking sheet using foil, and grease with cooking spray.
2. Stand the cabbage and run a knife from the top to bottom to cut the cabbage into wedges. Remove stems and wilted leaves. Mix the butter, garlic, salt, and black pepper until evenly combined.
3. Brush the mixture on every side of the cabbage wedges and sprinkle with Parmesan cheese.
4. Put on the baking sheet, then bake for at least 20 minutes to soften the cabbage and melt the cheese. Remove the cabbages when golden brown, plate, and sprinkle with extra cheese and parsley. Serve warm with pan-glazed tofu.

Nutrition:

- Calories: 268 kcal
- Fat: 19.3g
- Net Carbs: 4g
- Protein: 17.5g

52. Herb Pesto Tuna

Preparation Time: 10 minutes

Cooking Time: 10 minutes

Servings: 3

Ingredients:

- 3(3-ounce) yellowfin tuna fillets
- 1 tablespoon olive oil
- Freshly ground black pepper to taste
- ¼ cup Herb Pesto
- 1 lemon, cut into 8 thin slices

Directions:

1. Heat to medium - high barbecue. Add the olive oil to the fish and season each fillet with pepper. On the barbeque, cook it for 3 minutes. Turn over the fish and top each piece using the herb pesto and lemon slices. Grill until the tuna is cooked to medium-well for 5 to 6 minutes longer.
2. Modification of dialysis: The pesto adds to this recipe about 16 mg of potassium. The tuna is the reason why the potassium recipe is high. Try this recipe with other

fish like haddock or cod, but instead of putting it on the barbecue, broil the fish.

Nutrition:

- Fat: 2 g
- Phosphorus: 236 mg
- Sodium: 38 mg

53. Salmon and Coconut Mix

Preparation Time: 10 minutes

Cooking Time: 20 minutes

Servings: 4

Ingredients:

- 4 salmon fillets, boneless
- 3 tbsp. avocado mayonnaise
- 1 tsp. lime zest, grated
- ¼ cup coconut cream
- ¼ cup lime juice
- ½ cup coconut, unsweetened and shredded
- 2 tsp. Cajun seasoning
- A pinch of salt
- Pinch of black pepper

Directions:

1. Set the instant pot on Sauté mode, put the coconut cream and the rest of the ingredients except the fish, mix and cook for at least 5 minutes.
2. Add the fish, set the lid on, and cook on High for at least 10 minutes.
3. Release the pressure for 10 minutes, divide the salmon and sauce between plates and serve.

Nutrition:

- Calories 306 kcal
- Fat: 17.5g
- Fiber: 1.4g
- Carbs: 2.5g
- Protein: 25.3g

54. Buttery Scallops

Preparation Time: 10 minutes

Cooking Time: 10 minutes

Servings: 6

Ingredients:

- 2 pounds sea scallops
- 3 tablespoons butter, melted
- 2 tablespoons fresh thyme, minced
- Salt and pepper, to taste

Directions:

1. Preheat your air fryer to 390°F. Grease the air fryer cooking basket with butter.
2. Take a bowl, mix in all of the remaining ingredients, and toss well to coat the scallops.
3. Transfer scallops to air fryer cooking basket and cook for 5 minutes.
4. Repeat if any ingredients are left, serve, and enjoy!

Nutrition:

- Calories: 186 kcal
- Total Fat: 24g
- Total Carbs: 4g
- Fiber: 1g
- Net Carbs: 2g
- Protein: 20g

55. Old-Fashioned Turkey Chowder

Preparation Time: 15 minutes
Cooking Time: 35 minutes
Servings: 4

Ingredients:

- 2 tablespoons olive oil
- 2 tablespoons yellow onions, chopped
- 2 cloves garlic, roughly chopped
- ½ pound leftover roast turkey, shredded and skin removed
- 1 teaspoon Mediterranean spice mix
- 3 cups chicken bone broth
- 1 ½ cups milk
- ½ cup double cream
- 1 egg, lightly beaten
- 2 tablespoons dry sherry

Directions:

1. Heat the olive oil in a heavy-bottomed pot over a moderate flame. Sauté the onion and garlic until they've softened.
2. Stir in the leftover roast turkey, Mediterranean spice mix, and chicken bone broth; bring to a rapid boil. Partially cover and continue to cook for 20 to 25 minutes.
3. Turn the heat to simmer. Pour in the milk and double cream and continue to cook until it has reduced slightly.
4. Fold in the egg and dry sherry; continue to simmer, stirring frequently, for a further 2 minutes.

Nutrition:

- Calories: 350 kcal
- Fat: 25.8g
- Carbs: 5.5g
- Protein: 20g
- Fiber: 0.1g

57. Duck and Eggplant Casserole

Preparation Time: 10 minutes
Cooking Time: 45 minutes
Servings: 4

Ingredients:

- 1 pound ground duck meat
- 1 ½ tablespoons ghee, melted
- 1/3 cup double cream
- ½ pound eggplant, peeled and sliced
- 1 ½ cups almond flour
- Salt and black pepper, to taste
- ½teaspoon fennel seeds
- ½2 teaspoon oregano, dried
- 8 eggs

Directions:

1. Mix the almond flour with salt, black pepper, fennel seeds, and oregano. Fold in one egg and the melted ghee and whisk to combine well.

2. Press the crust into the bottom of a lightly-oiled pie pan. Cook the ground duck until no longer pink for about 3 minutes, stirring continuously.
3. Whisk the remaining eggs and double cream. Fold in the browned meat and stir until everything is well incorporated. Pour the mixture into the prepared crust. Top with the eggplant slices.
4. Bake for about 40 minutes. Cut into four pieces.

Nutrition:

- Calories: 562 kcal
- Fat: 49.5g
- Carbs: 6.7g
- Protein: 22.5g
- Fiber: 2.1g

58. Grated Cauliflower with Seasoned Mayo

Preparation Time: 10 minutes
Cooking Time: 15 minutes
Servings: 2

Ingredients:

- 1 pound grated cauliflower
- 3 oz. butter
- 4 eggs
- 3 oz. pimientos de padron or poblano peppers
- ½ cup mayonnaise
- 1 tsp. olive oil
- Salt and pepper to taste
- 1 tsp. garlic powder (optional)

Directions:

1. In a bowl, place the mayonnaise and garlic, then whisk and set aside.
2. Rinse, trim, then grate the cauliflower using a food processor or grater.
3. Melt a generous amount of butter and fry grated cauliflower for about 5 minutes. Season salt and pepper to taste.
4. Fry poblanos with oil until lightly crispy. Then fry eggs as you want and sprinkle salt and pepper over them.
5. Serve with poblanos and cauliflower. Drizzle some mayo mixture on top.

Nutrition:

- Calories: 898 kcal
- Fat: 87g
- Carbohydrates: 9g
- Protein: 17g

59. Paprika Roasted Radishes with Onions

Preparation Time: 20 minutes
Cooking Time: 20 minutes
Servings: 4

Ingredients:

- 2 large bunches radishes
- 1 small onion
- 2 tbsp. butter
- 2 tbsp. olive oil
- Tsp. fennel seeds
- ½ tsp. smoked paprika
- Sea salt and black pepper to taste

Directions:

1. Preheat the oven to 350°F. Line a rimmed preparing sheet with parchment paper.
2. In a blending bowl, combine radishes and onion. To the bowl, include spread, olive oil, fennel seeds, paprika, sea salt, and black pepper. Stir until radishes and onions are uniformly covered.
3. Pour radishes and onions in a solitary layer onto the parchment paper. Pour any additional spread and flavoring over the top.
4. Bake for 20 minutes.

Nutrition:

- Calories: 289 kcal
- Fat: 21.8g
- Carbs: 3.2g
- Protein: 12.3g

60. Yummy Garlic Chicken Livers

Preparation Time: 10 minutes
Cooking Time: 30 minutes
Servings: 2

Ingredients:

- ½ pound chicken liver
- 2 teaspoon lime juice
- 6 garlic cloves, mince
- ½ teaspoon salt
- 1 tbsp ginger garlic paste
- 1 cup diced onion
- 1 tbsp red chili powder
- 1 tsp cumin
- 1 tsp coriander powder
- Black pepper to taste
- 1 cardamom
- 2 tomatoes
- 1 cinnamon stick
- 1 bay leaf
- 4 tablespoon olive oil

Nutrition:

- Calories: 174 kcal
- Fats: 9g
- Protein: 18g
- Carbohydrates: 2.4g

Directions:

1. In a large pan, heat your oil over high heat.
2. Add the garlic and fry them golden brown.
3. Add onion and fry until they become caramelized.
4. Turn the heat to medium and add the bay leaf, cinnamon stick, cardamom and toss for 30 seconds.
5. Add the ginger garlic paste and 1 tbsp water. Adding water prevents burning.
6. Add the coriander powder, black pepper, salt, cumin, and red chili powder.
7. Cover and cook for 3 minutes on low heat.
8. Add the livers and cook on medium heat for 15 minutes.
9. Add the tomatoes and cook for another 5 minutes.
10. Check the seasoning, add more salt if needed.
11. Serve hot with tortilla.

21-DAY MEAL PLAN

DAYS	BREAKFAST	LUNCH	DINNER
1	Special Intermittent Bread	Intermittent Chicken Enchaladas	Parmesan Roasted Cabbage
2	Fried Eggs with Bacon	Pesto Pork Chops	Herb Pesto Tuna
3	Chicken Sausage Breakfast Casserole	Sausage and Cauliflower Rice	Salmon and Coconut Mix
4	Breakfast-Stuffed Bell Peppers	Double Cheese Meatloaf	Buttery Scallops
5	Small Intermittent Pies	Beef with Cabbage Noodles	Old-Fashioned Turkey Chowder
6	Intermittent Wraps	Roast Beef and Mozzarella Plate	Duck and Eggplant Casserole
7	Chicken Omelet	Sprouts Stir-fry with Kale, Broccoli, and Beef	Grated Cauliflower with Seasoned Mayo
8	Coconut Pancakes	Fennel & Figs Lamb	Paprika Roasted Radishes with Onions
9	Avocado Egg Bowls	Ground Beef and Cauliflower Hash	Cajun Chicken with Buckwheat Crust
10	Buttery Date Pancakes	Cheesy Taco Skillet	Healthy Mushroom and Arugula Pizza
11	Low Carb Pancake Crepes	Zoodle Soup with Italian Meatballs	Easy Mexican Casserole
12	Bacon Egg & Sausage Cups	Mini Thai Lamb Salad Bites	Stuffed Portobello Mushrooms
13	Cinnamon and Pecan Porridge	Smoked Salmon & Avocado Stacks	Quinoa and Turkey Stuffed Peppers

14	Chia Seed Banana Blueberry Delight	Sesame-Seared Salmon	Parmesan Roasted Cabbage
15	Morning Meatloaf	Spring Ramen Bowl	Herb Pesto Tuna
16	Savory Breakfast Muffins	Homemade Turkey Burger and Relish	Salmon and Coconut Mix
17	Low-Carb Brownies	Chicken Cobb Salad, With a BBQ Twist	Buttery Scallops
18	Apple Bread	Hearty Quinoa and Carrot Soup	Old-Fashioned Turkey Chowder
19	Coconut Protein Balls	Warming Lamb Stew	Duck and Eggplant Casserole
20	Protein Bars	Spicy Chicken Masala	Yummy Garlic Chicken Livers
21	Blueberry Muffins	Quick Ratatouille	Southwest Chicken Salad

This meal plan will make it easier to organize your meals, but of course, it can be adapted to the method you are following and your everyday life. In fact, in some cases, you may prefer to have only two meals. In this case, you can choose which one to skip, depending on your needs.

Conclusion

Thank you for reaching the end of this book on Intermittent Fasting for Women Over 50! I hope that through the pages of this book, you were able to gain the knowledge, understanding, and confidence you need to succeed with losing weight and gaining improved health.

While intermittent fasting may be an unorthodox lifestyle at this point, it was a standard and everyday part of life worldwide for centuries. Not only that, but science has proven it to be both safe and effective. There is no reason to hold back from this positive lifestyle proven through both time and science to be such an improvement. Whether you choose to practice intermittent fasting alone or with the ketogenic diet, you can expect to experience many benefits. While it may take a little time to adjust to the change in lifestyle, as all changes do, take heart in knowing that most people adjust and adapt within a month.

A healthy diet can be overwhelming, especially when shifting from a typical western diet of fast foods and sugar-loaded treatments. Being over 50 doesn't make it any easier. Nonetheless, after a few weeks on the fasting regiment, you will see an improvement in your mind, what you feel about yourself, your body and your life in general. Most individuals claim they have a lot of energy after practicing fasting for just a week or two.

The journey to an effective fasting system can be very challenging. Here are some rules for exploring this territory. Taking things one step at a time to understand the implications of the plan. Gradually pursue the fasting method. You just don't want to opt for something that may not be for you without thinking. You will continue fasting once every three weeks until you slowly change the time limit as you wish. For everyone, no system works the same way. Choose a scheme and configure it to suit your needs.

Decide whether it's good for you. Even after considering its many positive benefits, note that IF is not for everyone. The knowledge of nutrition and exercise will decide whether you can pursue it. If you are new to fitness and food, I strongly recommend that you first recognize the basics. Start slowly, smoothly, and gradually. If you decide you'd like to try IF, there's no rush. Pick one specific thing to try, even if it's a regular meal change of just one hour. Try this out and see how it works for you. Reflect on what IF strategies have in common, instead of going into too much detail. Sometimes you're feeding and sometimes you're not doing it. That pretty much sums it up.

Remember what's happening in your life. Consider how much preparation you're doing and how intensively you're practicing, how well you're going to rest and heal, how well IF blends into your daily practice or normal private activities, and what other stresses or life needs include. Note IF is one of the many forms of diet. But it is best only when it is regular, elastic, and part of your normal practice, not a task, and not a persistent physical and psychological pain source.

Know yourself and be informed about your interactions. Begin to collect data, gain knowledge, draw conclusions on yourself and your system, and direct future action. Do what's best for you. You are also supposed to give yourself time to adjust. Particularly because transitioning to your new program normally takes a few weeks. It is predicted that ups and downs will be present, but that is part of how life goes.

In this book, you were given all the information you need about intermittent fasting. Once you understand the way intermittent fasting works, it becomes easier to understand your body's metabolism. This diet works along with your metabolism to improve your overall health. Select a method of fasting that meets your needs and requirements. You don't have to make any drastic changes; you merely need to be mindful of when you eat. If you eat healthy and wholesome meals during the eating window, you will see an improvement in your overall health.

Thank you and good luck in your intermittent fasting journey.

Printed in Great Britain
by Amazon